# THE

# Alzheimer's

# Prevention

# Program

# THE
# Alzheimer's
# Prevention
# Program

## Keep Your Brain Healthy
## *for the* Rest *of* Your Life

# GARY SMALL, M.D.
DIRECTOR OF THE UCLA LONGEVITY CENTER
## & GIGI VORGAN
AUTHORS OF *THE MEMORY BIBLE*

WORKMAN PUBLISHING · NEW YORK

Copyright © 2011, 2012 by Gary Small, M.D., and Gigi Vorgan

Design copyright © by Workman Publishing
Photo copyright © by Gary Small, M.D.

Drawing of the woman's profile with the brain, courtesy of Diana Jacobs.
Photos of older senile brain and younger healthy brain courtesy of Harry Vinters, M.D.
Beatles photograph United Press International, 1964

The Library of Congress has cataloged the hardcover edition as follows:
Small, Gary W.
  The alzheimer's prevention program : keep your brain healthy for the rest of your life /
Gary Small, Gigi Vorgan.
      p. cm.
    ISBN 978-0-7611-6526-2 (hardback)
1. Alzheimer's disease--Prevention--Popular works. 2. Alzheimer's disease--Nutritional aspects--
Popular works. 3. Alzheimer's disease--Physiological aspects--Popular works.
I. Vorgan, Gigi, 1958- II. Title.
  RC523.2.S62 2012
  616.8'31--dc23
  2011025462

ISBN 978-0-7611-7222-2 (paperback)

Design by Lisa Hollander

Workman books are available at special discounts when purchased in bulk for premiums and
sales promotions as well as for fund-raising or educational use. Special editions of book excerpts
can also be created to specification. For details, contact the Special Sales Director at the address
below or send an email to specialmarkets@workman.com.

Workman Publishing Company, Inc.
225 Varick Street
New York, NY 10014-4381
workman.com

WORKMAN is a registered trademark of Workman Publishing Co., Inc.

Printed in the United States of America
First paperback printing November 2012

10 9 8 7 6 5 4 3 2

# Contents

# Acknowledgments

We are grateful to the volunteers and patients who participated in the many research studies that inspired this book. We also thank Diana Jacobs for her drawing of the human brain, Prabha Siddarth for her statistical input, our tireless and creative publicists Selina Meere and Courtney Greenhalgh, and our colleagues and friends who provided their guidance and input, including Susan Bowerman, Rachel Champeau, Mindy Gandin, Dr. Rob Gandin, Dr. David Heber, Jeffrey Nemerovsky, and Don Seigel. We are eternally thankful to our longtime agent and dear friend, Sandy Dijkstra, who has inspired our writing for many years; our talented publisher, Bob Miller; our gifted chief editor, Susan Bolotin; and our longtime friend and extraordinary editor, Mary Ellen O'Neill. This book would not have been possible without the love and support of our parents, Gertrude and Dr. Max Small and Rose and Fred Weiss, and our children, Rachel and Harry.

NOTE: The stories contained in this book are composite accounts based on the experiences of many individuals and do not represent any one person or group of people. Similarities to actual persons are coincidental and unintentional. Readers may wish to consult with their physician before initiating any diet or exercise program.

# Preface

For decades, researchers have been searching for a way to cure Alzheimer's disease, by far the most common cause of age-related mental decline. Despite considerable progress, no miracle remedy has yet been discovered.

But we don't need to sit and wait for a remarkable new drug or vaccine to come along before we start protecting our brains from this devastating disease. *The Alzheimer's Prevention Program* offers strategies to help delay symptoms from emerging. The scientific evidence points to prevention as today's most effective way to defend against Alzheimer's. If we can stave off the onset of dementia long enough for people never to experience symptoms in their lifetime—that in itself could be considered a cure.

Genetics accounts for only part of the risk for Alzheimer's disease, and we now know that lifestyle choices have a tremendous impact. A lifestyle that promotes brain health not only strengthens neurons and postpones mental decline, it also improves memory ability and brain efficiency right away. No matter where you are in your health profile—even if you exercise every day and eat all the right foods to keep your body and brain healthy—this program will still help you feel better and delay Alzheimer's disease longer. Whether you're a student, thirty-something, baby boomer, or senior, you will benefit quickly from practicing Alzheimer's prevention strategies—and you'll have fun doing it. It's never too early or too late to start protecting your brain. *The Alzheimer's Prevention Program* will show you how to get your brain healthy and do all you can to keep it that way for the rest of your life.

GARY SMALL, M.D., AND GIGI VORGAN
LOS ANGELES, CALIFORNIA, JANUARY 2012

"YOU CAN'T TURN BACK
THE CLOCK, BUT
YOU CAN WIND IT
UP AGAIN."

—BONNIE PRUDDEN,
PIONEER OF MYOTHERAPY

## CHAPTER 1

# Prevention Is Today's Best Defense

ONE EVENING MY WIFE, GIGI, AND I were leaving a restaurant when we spotted a well-known actress sitting at a table in the corner. We immediately recognized her, but we just couldn't come up with her name. As we walked toward the car, we tried prompting each other with what we *could* remember—leading men she'd worked with, a couple of her husbands, and that epic movie where she played a queen of England. We both felt so close to coming up with her name, but it just wouldn't pop into our brains. Finally, Gigi blurted out the actress's name. I asked how she was able to recall it, and she smugly reminded me that she was seven years younger than I.

She had a point. Age is the single greatest risk factor for developing memory loss. Most people over 40 begin to notice momentary recall delays and word-finding glitches similar to our tip-of-the-tongue experience at the restaurant. If the frequency of these experiences increases, it can be disconcerting, but it certainly doesn't mean that Alzheimer's disease is hovering in a dark corner. However, many of us still harbor a gnawing concern that our memory pauses could signal something more ominous.

In the U.S. nearly 80 million baby boomers, born between 1946 and 1964, are reaching the age when memory slips become more frequent, and they're concerned about it. Large-scale surveys show that more than 60 percent of middle-aged and older people have memory complaints, but only one out of five of them discusses these complaints with their doctor. Some may be frightened of what they could find out, or maybe they simply forget to tell.

Baby boomers are quite aware of the rising tide of Alzheimer's disease, perhaps the most overwhelming epidemic the world may ever see. Every 70 seconds, another American gets Alzheimer's disease, and by midcentury, a new case will develop every 30 seconds. Currently, 36 million people worldwide suffer from the disease. By 2050 we can expect 115 million cases of Alzheimer's, causing tremendous emotional distress and economic hardship.

The current wave of afflicted patients is already incurring a staggering price. In 2010 the estimated worldwide costs of medical and social care as well as informal care from unpaid family members and others totaled $604 billion. This figure accounts for approximately 1 percent of the world's gross domestic product. If caring for dementia were done by a company, its annual revenue would exceed that of Walmart.

## The Alzheimer's Fear Factor

A friend recently told me that after shopping at a large mall, he couldn't find his car in the lot. He could've sworn he had parked on level B, section 25, but he was obviously losing it. He felt his memory was going—and fast. A security guard drove him around the lot's several levels looking for his Mercedes, but he still couldn't find it. My friend started panicking. Maybe he wasn't just getting Alzheimer's, maybe he also had a brain tumor—malignant . . . Just then the security guard said they'd had several upscale cars stolen in the last month, many of them Mercedes. My friend almost cried with relief—his car had been stolen! Thank God!

Most baby boomers are terrified of Alzheimer's disease. Many have witnessed people in their parents' generation fall prey to its horrible effects. Some have endured the helplessness and pain of watching someone they love gradually fade away.

But today's proactive boomers don't plan to sit back and take it. They grew up during the tumultuous '60s and '70s and have no qualms about facing a challenge and testing conventional wisdom. As they've aged, many baby boomers have embraced the concept that an active lifestyle can keep them feeling healthy and young. They know about the research confirming that the same lifestyle choices that protect the body also protect the mind. Physical exercise, a nutritious diet, mental stimulation, and stress reduction have their greatest impact when people combine these strategies and continue them for several years.

## Taking Control of Your Brain Health

A s these millions of baby boomers approach age 65, when their risk for Alzheimer's disease begins to accelerate, are they all headed for disaster? Are they facing an inevitable future of mental decline and dementia? The answer is a definitive no. We *do* have the ability to influence our future brain health, and we are not all destined to experience a precipitous fall into mental fog. Science has shown that genetics, our hereditary predisposition for Alzheimer's disease, accounts for only part of our risk: Lifestyle choices may have an even greater impact. Therefore, we have more control than we think.

One of my neighbors mentioned to me that he was amazed by how many Alzheimer's articles there were in the newspapers these days. He'd read all about these new research findings, yet he was still confused. Should he have a spinal tap or brain PET scan to see if he was going to get the disease? And if the tests turned out positive, what could he do? Could drugs really make a difference? And what about this diet I'd been talking about for protecting the brain; should he crank up his Sudoku level to diabolical? Was jogging a mile every day better than swimming ten laps? He finally confessed that when he does try doing something to protect his brain, he usually doesn't feel any different and after a few days he gets distracted and stops. And playing those boring computer brain games was worse than shopping with his wife.

My neighbor is not alone. A lot of people are confused about what all the latest scientific information means and how it applies to their own lives. *The Alzheimer's Prevention Program* will clear up much of the confusion and provide an easy-to-follow plan of action to improve memory ability now and optimize your brain health for the future.

The greatest challenge for people like my neighbor lies in getting started and sticking with a healthy brain lifestyle for the long haul. One thing I've learned through my medical practice and research experience in the past three decades is that an effective Alzheimer's prevention program not only has to begin improving memory and mental acuity quickly, but it also has to be fun and easy to use. When people notice benefits right away, it motivates them to change their behaviors, which then become new healthy habits.

*The Alzheimer's Prevention Program* will spell out exactly what you need to do for your first seven days. In that time, you will see for yourself how easy it is to achieve positive results. The book will also clarify the controversies and conflicting discoveries about Alzheimer's disease and explain the scientific evidence that shows how we can best defend ourselves against it.

## What Is Alzheimer's Disease?

In 1906 Alois Alzheimer presented the first report of the disease that was later named after him. At a gathering of fellow German psychiatrists, he described a 51-year-old woman who developed confusion, memory loss, and psychotic symptoms that rapidly progressed until she died four years later. Dr. Alzheimer applied chemical stains to brain tissue obtained during her autopsy. When he viewed thin slices of the tissue under the microscope, he could see tiny amyloid plaques and tau tangles—the abnormal waxy protein fragments and twisted fibers that define the disease. These microscopic deposits were scattered throughout her brain, especially in areas that control memory and other mental functions such as language, decision making, and personality.

Although this discovery was one of the first to connect a specific physical brain abnormality to a mental disorder, the medical community didn't pay much attention to it for more than fifty years, because Alzheimer's disease was considered an extremely rare condition afflicting only a few unfortunate middle-aged people with presenile dementia. Doctors believed senility was just a normal part of aging. When people got old enough, they weren't expected to remember much, and their aging brains atrophied. Scientists showed during autopsy that the brain of an older senile individual had become smaller and had deeper crevices compared with a younger person's brain, as seen on page 16.

In the late 1960s, however, neuropathologists systematically studied these older senile brains after autopsy, using the same chemical dyes that Dr. Alzheimer used. They spotted those same tiny waxy plaques and tangled threads of tau protein in brains of people who had died from the very common senile dementia, a condition that seemed to afflict nearly all seniors if they lived long enough. In fact, the older senile brains were filled with plaques and tangles. Because of these studies, this type of senility was finally termed Alzheimer's disease.

After that, an epidemic of Alzheimer's disease was declared and the world recognized that the senility that grandma and grandpa got when they reached 70 or older was not just a regular part of aging. It was a disease attacking their brain cells—a buildup of sticky proteins that caused neurons to misfire, mucking up their signals.

No one knew how to stop the disease's relentless infiltration throughout the brains of these patients. They did know, however, that amyloid plaques and tau tangles initially emerged from deep structures in the brain's temporal lobe (beneath the temples) and then spread throughout its outer rim, or cortex, first attacking cells that control short-term memory while long-term memory remained preserved: A patient with mild Alzheimer's disease may recall her pals from high school but forget what she ate for lunch. As the disease progresses, unfortunately, the patient may not only forget the names of close relatives, but her ability to reason and make sound judgments will begin to slip: She can no longer manage her finances or find her way home from the market. Many patients experience noticeable changes in personality—the core of what defines them as an individual. Sometimes an exaggeration of their preexisting personality traits can be the first sign of brain degeneration.

I evaluated a successful entrepreneur who had become wealthy through his daring and unusual investment choices. His family eventually brought him to see me because his investment strategies were now losing money and eroding the family fortune, but he wouldn't take advice from anyone. They also noticed a change in his personality from his usual gregarious and engaging self to someone who had few interpersonal boundaries: He would walk up to strangers on the street and give them financial advice. In fact, during our first meeting, he asked me to go into business with him on a windmill company.

It turned out that he had a dementia that attacked the frontal and temporal lobes of his brain. He may have had symptoms for years, but while he was making money, nobody questioned his mental capacity even though he often acted strangely. After an extensive medical evaluation, I started him on a medication regimen that brought more control to his frontal lobe, which helped with his executive decision-making problems and volatile personality. Like many of my patients who already have dementia, I was able to combine medical treatments with the Alzheimer's program lifestyle strategies. Thanks to the medication, his personal relationships improved, which lowered his stress levels and helped him remain organized enough to exercise every day and stay on a healthy brain diet. Although he did pretty well for the next year, eventually his cognitive abilities worsened, and he took his family's advice and retired. I've heard that the windmill company I passed on became a huge success.

## The New Science of Alzheimer's Prevention

Most people know that the course of the illness is bleak; however, recent discoveries are encouraging about future treatments. The latest research is also clarifying what is really going on in the brain as it ages, offering us more opportunities to stave off the effects of Alzheimer's disease for years.

When I discuss prevention strategies with people, occasionally someone will ask whether there is a proven cure or prevention for Alzheimer's disease. A recent National Institutes of Health (NIH) consensus panel couldn't draw firm conclusions regarding the relationship between decreasing risk factors for Alzheimer's disease and slowing cognitive decline. However, the panel did say that many studies of healthy lifestyle habits—including diet, physical activity, and cognitive engagement—are providing new insights into the prevention of cognitive decline and Alzheimer's disease.

I certainly agree with the panel's call for additional studies to supplement these findings, but since these lifestyle choices help us feel better right away and appear to help prevent several diseases that increase Alzheimer's risk, why wait? I and many other experts agree: Why not get started on an Alzheimer's prevention program while we wait for the results of large-scale definitive studies, which could take decades to complete?

I recently gave a lecture to a group of doctors about how the amyloid plaques and tau tangles of Alzheimer's disease begin accumulating in our brains as early as our twenties and thirties. I noticed a young woman in the front row squirming in her seat. She jumped up from her chair as soon as the lecture ended and ambushed me with a question about her age-related memory challenges. She was having trouble keeping track of her patients' conditions and more than occasionally misplaced her car keys and glasses. She had no family history of Alzheimer's disease, but after hearing my lecture, she felt sure that she was getting it. I asked her if she was under a lot of stress and she laughed. "Trust me, Dr. Small—cardiac surgery is no picnic for a woman. I haven't had time to do a triathlon for over a year, and I'm turning thirty-four next month."

**TRY THIS!**

To warm up your neural circuits, close your eyes and sign your name as neatly as possible. Check out your penmanship and see if you get better on your second try.

This 34-year-old triathlete/surgeon turned out to be one of what is often called "the worried well"—people who are anxious about non-existent diagnoses. As I suspected, her worries about having early-onset Alzheimer's disease symptoms were unfounded, but her stress level was very high, and stress is one of the major causes of forgetfulness. Some people—even doctors—get extremely anxious when they learn that the tiny amyloid plaques and tau tangles that contribute to Alzheimer's disease can be detected in the brains of healthy people as young as age 30.

When neuropathologists looked at hundreds of autopsied brains from people who died at various ages, they found only a few scattered plaques and tangles in people who died in their 20s; but in the brains of people who died a decade older, they found more. In fact, the studies revealed a significant correlation between the age of a healthy brain and the number of Alzheimer's plaques and tangles it contained. Also, the pattern of distribution of these abnormal deposits was consistent with Alois Alzheimer's early findings indicating that the disease begins in specific memory centers deep within the brain and then spreads to other memory and thinking regions in the brain's outer rim or cortex.

Until just the last decade, autopsy studies of the brain were the only way that Alzheimer's disease could be confirmed. But in 2002, our UCLA research team discovered a new way of using a PET (positron emission tomography) scan of the brain that allowed us to visualize the tiny plaques and tangles of Alzheimer's disease in living patients for the first time. The same areas showing high concentrations of amyloid plaques and tau tangles at autopsy lit up brightly in our FDDNP (a radioactive tracer) PET scans of patients with the disease.

Since this initial discovery, we have studied hundreds of people ranging from their 20s to their 90s, and these volunteers and patients all have varying degrees of brain aging and memory decline. Some have moderate to severe Alzheimer's symptoms, while others show no symptoms at all. Our studies confirmed what pathologists had reported earlier in their autopsy investigations: Plaques and tangles begin to build up in the brain decades before any symptoms of Alzheimer's emerge.

Like the young surgeon who attended my lecture, people often become frightened when they first hear about this discovery. They often don't want to get a brain scan because they fear that once their brains have plaques and tangles, it's too late to slow or halt the process. In truth, though, the discovery is tremendously powerful. It offers us the opportunity to identify people at risk very early in the course of their brain aging, so they can begin preventive strategies and lifestyle programs to protect their healthy neurons rather than wait for some possible future treatment that might repair damaged ones.

Nearly all of us have some plaques and tangles in our brains, but they don't begin to affect us until the accumulation reaches a critical threshold—a tipping point when our brains can no longer compensate for the misfiring neurons. Scientists have come up with new terminology to better categorize the degree of brain aging and neural degeneration that affect people at various stages of life, and these categories have been helpful in studying medicines and other interventions in people at risk for dementia or mental impairment that interferes with their daily life.

## Mild Cognitive Impairment: A Transition Phase

Occasionally, friends get worried about a relative's memory loss, but the relative becomes defensive or says that's ridiculous and refuses to come in for an evaluation. Recently Gigi and I went to dinner at the home of her friend, who was concerned that her 82-year-old father, Mel, was getting Alzheimer's disease. I sat next to him during a two-hour dinner and did an informal assessment. During dinner Mel often repeated himself and sometimes had trouble finding words and recalling details, but he did follow the conversation. He had a pretty good sense of humor and even laughed at some of my lame jokes. There were a few moments when he stared off into space, as if he was either thinking thoughts all his own or no thoughts at all, but those were very brief.

I chatted with Mel's wife over coffee, and she told me that he still likes going to the market for her and balances their checkbook just fine. I didn't think he had Alzheimer's disease, but he was somewhere on the road to getting it. Now that Mel had met me, he agreed to come in to the office with his wife. They both got started on the Alzheimer's Prevention Program, and I prescribed Aricept for Mel, an antidementia medicine that sometimes delays the onset of Alzheimer's disease. Even in your eighties, it's not too late to begin protecting your brain.

Dr. Ron Petersen of the Mayo Clinic introduced the term *mild cognitive impairment,* or MCI, which is often defined as a memory impairment that is similar to what we see in very mild Alzheimer's disease. MCI patients are still independent and can manage daily functioning, whereas patients with Alzheimer's dementia need help from others. However, if I tried to teach ten new words to someone with MCI—perhaps said the words slowly several times—that person might remember only three or four of them after a ten-minute pause. He might remember a couple more by practicing some simple memory techniques, but he still probably would not do as well as the average individual in his age group who did not have MCI. Compared to someone who ages normally, people with this kind of MCI have a ten to fifteen times higher risk of developing Alzheimer's disease each year.

In the figure below, we can see the trajectory of one patient's mental decline as he develops Alzheimer's disease. MCI is a transition phase between normal aging (including middle-age forgetfulness) and the more significant impairment observed in Alzheimer's dementia.

Scientists have already begun testing anti-Alzheimer's medications in people with MCI to see if it's possible to delay the onset of Alzheimer's symptoms, but the results have not always been conclusive. One difficulty with the diagnosis of MCI is that as time passes, some patients remain stable, a few improve, and many experience cognitive decline. New brain scanning and biomarker technologies are helping us sort out these subgroups of MCI patients for testing both medications and brain-protective lifestyle strategies. Some of the diagnostic techniques are so sensitive and

## MENTAL FUNCTION VS. AGE

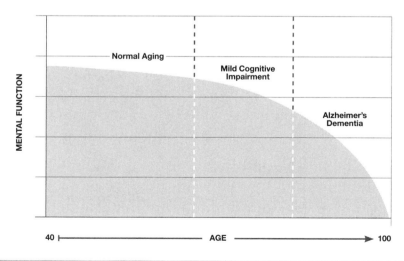

specific that they can even identify people who are aging normally but may be at higher risk for developing MCI. These methods allow us to look at the underlying biology of the brain so we don't need to rely completely on standardized paper-and-pencil tests that assess memory and other mental abilities. These new research tools have led many leading scientists throughout the world to redefine Alzheimer's disease itself.

Experts have revised the definitions for Alzheimer's disease to include people who have MCI along with positive PET-scan or spinal-tap test results for plaques and tangles. So those with MCI and an amyloid-positive biomarker test are now considered to have a mild form of Alzheimer's disease, and amyloid-positive people with normal aging who merely have small numbers of plaques and tangles in their brains are now considered to have preclinical Alzheimer's disease. These plaques and tangles build up in the brain of every individual at a different rate depending on lifestyle and genetic predisposition. Does that mean we will all eventually get Alzheimer's disease if we live long enough? Perhaps so, but many people won't experience any symptoms until they reach 110 years of age or older, and few people live that long.

Mme. Jeanne Calment of France was free of Alzheimer's disease when she died at 122, but what if she had lived to 132 or 140? It's very possible that her brain would have accumulated enough plaques and tangles to disrupt her memory and thinking. It's interesting to note that Madame Calment was an astute businesswoman. At age 94, she sold her attractive Arles apartment to a French investor under a contract that allowed her to stay there rent-free for the rest of her life. *He* died ten years later.

## Genetics: Living by the Code

Just as we can't choose our parents, we can't choose our genetics—although I know people who would very much like to have some say in both those choices. Scientists are working hard in stem cell research, conducting cloning studies and other experiments in an attempt to significantly alter our genetic makeup, but the practical applications from these studies are still a long way off.

With Alzheimer's disease, no one knows precisely if or when symptoms will strike during their lifetime. In rare situations, a genetic mutation or error in the DNA of a family causes a cluster of cases in middle-aged relatives. In these uncommon families (less than 3 percent of all patients), genetic testing can determine which half of the relatives will develop the disease early in life. Many members of these families consult with genetic counselors and decide whether they want to be tested for an Alzheimer's mutation so they can plan for the future. This knowledge, however, affects people in different ways psychologically. For example, one person with an Alzheimer's genetic mutation may enthusiastically embrace a brain-protective healthy lifestyle to forestall symptoms as long as possible; another might become severely depressed, which can worsen memory loss and accelerate cognitive decline. Occasionally, a relative who tests negative for a genetic mutation may experience survivor guilt and therefore get depressed.

More than 99 percent of us don't have to worry about Alzheimer's genetic mutations because we don't have a family history of early-onset Alzheimer's disease (before age 65). Usually, if Alzheimer's does strike a family, it tends to affect only a few relatives, late in life.

One out of every five people in the general population, however, does carry a common genetic variant, or allele, known as APOE-4. This is not a genetic mutation, so it doesn't actually cause the disease; it is only a variant of a gene that increases an individual's risk for getting Alzheimer's disease after age 65, but it is far from a sure thing. People who have the APOE-4 gene may never get Alzheimer's; conversely, others who don't carry APOE-4 may get Alzheimer's disease anyway.

I participated in a national consensus conference not long after the initial APOE-4 discovery was made. The experts there concluded that doctors should dissuade patients from APOE-4 testing as a diagnostic predictor, because of the potential negative psychological consequences. However, the psychological effects of this genetic knowledge had not

Q: **Is it true that people whose mothers had Alzheimer's disease are at greater risk than if their fathers had it?**

A: Scientists at New York University recently studied the brain scans of unaffected people whose parents had Alzheimer's. In these adult children, the likelihood of subtle declines in brain function was significantly greater in those whose mothers suffered from the disease than those whose fathers did. The details of how this kind of inheritance occurs and the extent of its effect on an individual's risk for the disease have not yet been determined.

been studied systematically, and not all the experts agreed.

Years later, Dr. Robert Green and colleagues at Boston University finally did do a study addressing this issue. They found that when people received a positive result on their APOE-4 test and understood that it didn't mean they were surely destined to get the disease, they became no more depressed than people who received negative results. My own UCLA research has shown that many APOE-4 carriers who learn of their genetic risk become the most enthusiastic followers of this Alzheimer's Prevention Program.

The bottom line is that our DNA does not tell the whole story. The MacArthur Study of Successful Aging taught us an important lesson: If we define successful aging as physical *and* mental health, then genetics is responsible for only a third of the formula for how long and how well we live. The other two thirds are nongenetic, and the lifestyle choices we make every day may be the biggest factor in preventing Alzheimer's disease.

This became particularly clear when our UCLA group studied several sets of identical twins in their 80s with exactly the same genetic makeup. One twin got Alzheimer's while the other twin—who had led a healthier life—either never got the disease or else developed symptoms much later in life.

## Plaque: Foe or No?

I think I read maybe one paragraph in my medical school pathology textbook that referred to amyloid plaques and tau tangles. And I recall looking at perhaps one or two slides of an autopsied Alzheimer's brain showing the deposits. I had no idea that decades later, plaques and tangles would be a hotly debated scientific topic. In 2010 I moderated a panel of Alzheimer's experts at a national meeting concerning alternatives to the amyloid hypothesis. My e-mail server was filled with correspondence from frustrated scientists who couldn't get their fringe theories included in the debate.

When it comes to amyloid plaques and tau tangles and how much they contribute to Alzheimer's disease, scientists have been engaged in a heated controversy for years. To confirm the diagnosis of the disease, the brain has to have high levels of these abnormal protein deposits, and some researchers are convinced that their gradual accumulation is the primary cause of the disease. Other investigators argue that plaques and tangles are just markers of the disease and not the cause. These scientists see the plaques and tangles as scattered debris of the disease, which they suspect may be caused by some other process, perhaps a misfiring of brain neurons, general inflammation, genetic malfunction, or some other mechanical breakdown. These alternative theories might explain why some of the latest studies of antiplaque treatments have failed. Removing the amyloid plaques from the brain may have as limited an effect on the disease as taking an aspirin for a fever when the patient really needs antibiotics to treat the underlying infection causing the fever.

In support of the latter argument, researchers have discovered tiny proteins, called oligomers, which are toxic to brain cells. These oligomers are the precursors or building blocks of the insoluble amyloid plaques. If a novel drug were able to clear out the plaques and tangles in a brain, the deposits might simply return because they may be continuously building up from those pesky little oligomers.

Another possibility is that amyloid buildup is only one aspect of the problem. Since the accumulation of tau tangles in the brain corresponds much more closely to the progression of memory decline, some experts contend that the tau tangles, not the amyloid plaques, should be the main target of new drug development. So far, there haven't been many drugs in development to eliminate or clear out just the tau tangles.

## Angry, Rusty Brains

Not long ago I received a 12-page handwritten letter from a school-teacher in Australia who was convinced that scented shampoo somehow penetrated the blood–brain barrier and was the cause of Alzheimer's. Another e-mail implicated the diminishing ozone layer's allowing radiation from outer space to cause neuronal dysfunction and ultimately Alzheimer's disease. I'm always game to explore a new theory, but I prefer to focus on those based on more substantial science.

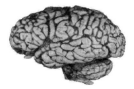

YOUNGER HEALTHY BRAIN: A healthy brain shows no sign of inflammation or atrophy.

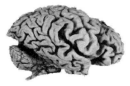

OLDER SENILE BRAIN: The kind of aging and atrophy shown in this brain was formerly believed to be normal, but in fact showed signs of inflammation and decline.

Beyond the plaque and tangle controversy, many controlled studies implicate other brain malfunctions that could lead to dementia. For example, inflammation and oxidation appear to contribute to the progression of Alzheimer's disease, just as they do in heart disease, diabetes, cancer, and aging itself.

Inflammation is usually a health-promoting process: It prompts the body to respond to injury and irritation. One might experience inflammation as pain, swelling, redness, and heat, as in arthritis—what some doctors describe as an *angry* joint. At a cellular level, inflammation can mean that the body is attacking a foreign object, irritation, or infection, which leads the way toward healing a wound or killing off the offending bacterium or virus.

When scientists looked more closely at the amyloid plaques in Alzheimer's brains, they discovered evidence of inflammation, including cytokines (very tiny protein molecules that attack foreign material) and activated microglia (minute cells that clean out cellular waste in the central nervous system, ridding it of damaged neurons, plaques, and infectious agents). Inflammation is generally a good thing, signifying that the body is working to heal itself, but sometimes too much of a good thing is not good for us. One theory is that chronic inflammation in the brain destroys neurons. Other studies have found a link between better brain health and medicines, foods, and lifestyle choices that reduce inflammation in the body.

Oxidation is a process that can be observed in the browning of sliced fruit or the rusting of a bicycle left outdoors. In our bodies, oxidation is necessary for our cells to do their work, but the process results in byproducts known as oxidants or free radicals. Like all the body's cells, brain cells undergo wear and tear from these free radicals, which can damage the genetic material of otherwise healthy cells. This oxidative stress accelerates nearly all age-related diseases from cancer to cataracts to Alzheimer's. Eating antioxidant fruits and vegetables to combat oxidation is a critical component of a diet that protects us from Alzheimer's disease.

## The Three Most Important Words in Alzheimer's Prevention

Most of us know the three most important words in real estate: location, location, location. But how many of us know the three most important words in Alzheimer's prevention? Timing, timing, timing.

A particular brain-protective treatment that is effective at one point in time can be less effective if we wait too long to use it. In fact, some therapies may even be harmful if the timing is slightly off. The most effective point in time for using a certain treatment may be years, even decades, before any symptoms of mental decline are noticeable. At later stages, different treatments may be called for.

An example of how treatment timing can be critical is the use of anti-inflammatory medicines. Many doctors first got interested in the possibility that inflammation might be involved in brain aging when they learned about the results of the Baltimore Longitudinal Study.

Nondemented study volunteers who took common anti-inflammatory drugs, including ibuprofen (Motrin) and naproxen (Aleve), for two or more years had a 60 percent lower risk for developing Alzheimer's disease in the future.

Although the study included a large number of subjects, it didn't prove a definitive cause and effect between taking the drugs and defending against Alzheimer's. To look at that issue more directly, my UCLA research team conducted a double-blind study in middle-aged people with very mild memory complaints when there were relatively few amyloid plaques and tau tangles in their brains. In this NIH-funded study, we compared the anti-inflammatory drug celecoxib (Celebrex) to a placebo and found that people who took the active drug for 18 months had higher brain activity in the frontal lobe, a region controlling memory and complex reasoning. They also had better scores on several memory tests. The placebo group did not show these gains.

Dr. John Breitner and his coworkers at the University of Washington, however, found that anti-inflammatory treatments can be harmful to the brain when used later in the course of brain aging, when people reach their 70s and begin to experience more severe cognitive symptoms. In fact, in patients with Alzheimer's dementia—when plaques and tangles are highly concentrated in their brains—these same anti-inflammatory drugs appear to accelerate mental decline. It may be that the drugs control brain inflammation and protect neurons in middle age, but once too many plaques and tangles accumulate in the brain, they somehow damage the neurons. Another issue is the amount of medicine that actually gets into the brain. Once Alzheimer's disease causes symptoms, the blood–brain barrier (a

Q: I have heard that some people have their dental fillings replaced or removed to avoid Alzheimer's. What's that about?

A: For many years people have expressed concern that the mercury and other toxins from dental fillings may get into the blood system and cause damage that contributes to various health problems ranging from chronic fatigue syndrome to Alzheimer's disease. Several large-scale studies, one including more than 20,000 people, have failed to confirm any significant association between dental fillings and Alzheimer's disease.

protective membrane that separates circulating blood from brain cells) starts leaking, so the brain is exposed to greater amounts of the drug, which could be toxic to neurons.

We don't have enough information yet about the timing and dosing of anti-inflammatory medicines to make specific recommendations about when and how they might be used to defend against mental decline. I am certainly not suggesting that everyone run out and start popping Motrin as if it were the new Alzheimer's preventive or cure. These medicines have potentially dangerous side effects, such as elevated blood pressure, possible internal bleeding, and even kidney failure, and our study was too small to definitively prove effectiveness. If you are already taking an anti-inflammatory drug for joint pain or some other illness, it may well be protecting your brain, but before you begin taking a medicine, always discuss the side effects with your doctor.

A healthy lifestyle that includes physical exercise and good nutrition can reduce inflammation throughout the body and the brain, and it has no detrimental side effects. Of course, you could twist your ankle on a power walk, but when you exercise in moderation and increase your intensity slowly, you become stronger and less likely to incur injuries. The Alzheimer's prevention physical fitness program combines strengthening exercises, cardiovascular conditioning, and balance and stability training. This approach to exercise will not only protect your brain but also increase your heart health and possibly extend your lifespan.

## The Power of a Strong Defense

In football the object of the defensive team is to prevent its opponents from scoring. The object of an Alzheimer's prevention program is to push back the offensive assault of the disease. And just as in football, Alzheimer's prevention can be very aggressive and may determine the outcome of the game. If your defensive team is tough enough, it may stave off the symptoms of the disease for your lifetime.

Alzheimer's disease is one of many age-related illnesses that so far have no permanent cure to eradicate the underlying cause. Like some cancers, diabetes, high cholesterol, and hypertension, it begins in middle age or later, worsens with time, and if left untreated, significantly diminishes one's quality of life and shortens life expectancy.

For most age-related illnesses, doctors usually determine an individual's disease risk or severity using biomarkers: numeric measures including blood pressure, blood cholesterol, or blood sugar. Patients at risk for these illnesses usually remain on treatments for several years with the goal of keeping the disease measure at a low level, which minimizes their future risk for worsening of disease, whether it's stroke, a heart attack, or diabetes. Occasionally an age-related disease can be completely eradicated or cured, for instance when a surgeon removes an isolated tumor. More often with cancer, a patient receives several treatments (e.g., radiation, chemotherapy, and surgery), and if the cancer does not recur within five years, most doctors consider the patient cured.

I'm optimistic that we will eventually discover a definitive cure for Alzheimer's disease that is as effective as an antibiotic for an infection. For now, though, the most promising path is through prevention—protecting a healthy brain rather than trying to reverse neural damage that has already occurred. Considerable scientific evidence points to lifestyle as key to defending our brains from Alzheimer's disease. Diet, mental and physical exercise, stress reduction, social engagement—these and other strategies not only improve cognitive performance quickly, but they may also delay the onset of dementia for many people. Although some experts have called for additional long-term studies, most baby boomers aren't willing to sit around and wait 30 years for

Q: **Do women have a greater risk for dementia than men do?**

A: The answer depends on your age and the type of dementia. One of the largest systematic studies to address this question did not find any difference in the incidence of dementia between women and men ages 55 to 90 years. However, after age 90 the incidence of Alzheimer's disease went down slightly for men but not for women. At any age, men were more likely to develop vascular dementia. The explanation for these differences is not clear, but it relates to both biological factors and lifestyle behaviors such as smoking.

definitive study results before starting to protect their brains. We already know that many of these lifestyle strategies help maintain heart health, lower the risk for diabetes, and quickly improve memory and cognitive abilities.

Proactive healthy brain lifestyles offer an opportunity to have a major public health impact. In our UCLA collaboration with the RAND Corporation think tank, we reviewed the most reliable epidemiological studies showing that healthy lifestyle behaviors lower the risk for Alzheimer's, then calculated how much each behavior may delay the onset of dementia symptoms. From that analysis, we concluded that if everyone in the U.S. adopted just one additional healthy lifestyle habit (perhaps took a brisk walk every other day or ate fish twice a week), within five years we could anticipate one million fewer cases of Alzheimer's disease than otherwise expected. Additional studies suggest that if we engaged in more than one healthy lifestyle habit we could possibly delay the onset of Alzheimer's even more. In fact, an estimated six million people expected to develop the disease by 2050 might be spared, and the nation could save nearly $300 billion.

## How Long May Prevention Forestall Alzheimer's?

We can estimate the potential impact of a healthy lifestyle program on our risk for Alzheimer's disease by looking at previous studies that have demonstrated a connection between lifestyle habits and future risk for the disease. From these results, we can assume that spending time engaged in such habits may delay the onset of symptoms for a certain number of years. A recent study indicated that physical exercise several times a week over a two-year period lowered a person's future risk for memory decline by 46 percent. Eating antioxidant fruits and vegetables such as blueberries and broccoli for a four-year period reduced dementia risk by 44 percent. People who spend time doing complex mental tasks during midlife decreased their dementia risk by as much as 48 percent.

21

## TWO-YEAR DELAY IN ONSET OF SYMPTOMS

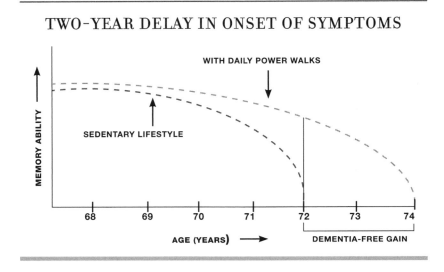

My patient Jack W., a 62-year-old foundation president, was glued to his office computer all day, then went home and sat in front of his laptop all evening. Although he was a smart man engaged in an intellectual pursuit, he wasn't getting any exercise at all. If Jack continued his couch-potato lifestyle—spending all his leisure time munching on chips in front of the computer—then according to his genetic predisposition, he would begin developing dementia symptoms by age 72.

When I reviewed Jack's risk factors for dementia with him, he finally turned off the computer and got up from his chair. He started walking with a buddy five mornings a week. Previous studies connecting regular physical exercise with reduced Alzheimer's risk indicated that if Jack continued his walks for four years, the onset of his dementia symptoms would be delayed until the age of 74, although it could be delayed longer and his dementia symptoms may be milder.

The estimate of a two-year delay in dementia onset may be conservative. In fact, once Jack got into it, he looked forward to walking with his friend—they had a lot of laughs, bragged about their grandkids, and

## FOUR-YEAR DELAY IN ONSET OF SYMPTOMS

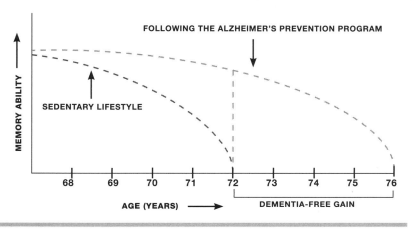

Jack reported a lift in his mood. He began to manage stress better at work and even lost a few pounds.

So now Jack was doing more than just walking. He was following other Alzheimer's prevention lifestyle suggestions as well. He had become more socially engaged, which lowered his stress levels. His weight loss had inspired him to toss out the chips and add fresh fruits and vegetables to his daily diet, along with fish twice a week. If we add up the effect of his two new lifestyle routines, exercising and healthy eating, then Jack's Alzheimer's symptoms could be staved off for an additional year, until age 75.

Jack stuck to his Alzheimer's prevention program for more than four years. In fact, it became his permanent lifestyle. He practiced mental aerobics and did crosswords—even Friday puzzles—in pen. If we add in the effects of his improved social life, stress management, and mental stimulation, then his anticipated dementia-free years increased to a total of four, so his expected age of dementia onset was pushed back to age 76.

Jack was doing so well that he no longer came to see me regularly, but he did keep in touch over the years. He retired on his 70th birthday and traveled frequently with his wife. When Jack turned 75, he came in for a checkup, concerned about his occasional memory slips. I found no evidence of dementia, not even mild cognitive impairment. Jack's Alzheimer's prevention strategies had made a big difference in his life, allowing him to remain active and Alzheimer's-free for several extra years. And Jack didn't even start his prevention plan until he was in his 60s.

## One Plus One Equals Three

We all know that physical exercise, stress reduction, healthy nutrition, and memory training are good for our brains, but people may not realize that combining these strategies creates a synergy that has a greater impact than just doing one or two of the strategies on their own. For our initial UCLA healthy brain lifestyle study, we kept the psychologist who was doing the assessments as unbiased as possible by not telling her which volunteers followed the "intervention" and which ones did not. After two weeks, she was amazed because the memory scores of half the volunteers had shot up dramatically. She wanted to know if this drug we were testing was on the market yet and whether she could get some. When I explained to her that we were not testing a drug but instead a program of lifestyle strategies and exercises, she insisted on getting a copy of the program and wanted to get started that day.

This kind of enthusiasm is common. When people see quick positive results, they become true believers and advocates of an Alzheimer's prevention program. Systematic studies have documented these positive outcomes—including memory improvement, increased energy levels, less stress and better mood. Volunteers also report having more confidence, sleeping better, and even losing weight without trying.

Other studies have reported similar kinds of synergy from combining multiple healthy lifestyle habits. A healthy diet combined with regular physical exercise reduced the risk for diabetes. Another strategy integrating stress reduction with physical activity was shown to lower the risk of chest pain in cardiac patients compared with exercise alone. Dietary change, aerobic exercise, and smoking cessation regimens raised good HDL cholesterol levels, and when combined with medication or vitamin therapy, the effects were amplified further. People learning memory techniques along with following a physical exercise regimen tended to get better sleep, which further increased their focus and memory ability.

## Building Brain Muscle

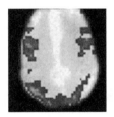

fMRI before

A 51-year-old nurse at a local hospital, Helen G., constantly joked about her multitasking problems and memory slips, but behind the humor I sensed her fear and anxiety. The last straw for her was the day she forgot to pick her daughter up from soccer practice. Helen was convinced that she had serious memory problems and was eager to volunteer for our study. She told me that several of her relatives had gotten Alzheimer's disease in their 80s, and admitted that she got scared every time she misplaced a file or forgot a patient's name.

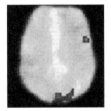

fMRI after

Before entering the study, she underwent a brain stress test: While we measured her brain activity in a functional MRI (fMRI) scanner, we read her a list of unrelated word pairs like "apple phone" or "umbrella baseball." After a pause, she tried to recall the word pairs she had just heard. The upper image is an MRI picture of what her brain stress test looked like at baseline, before any healthy brain intervention.

The dark areas show where her brain was active while she tried to recall the word pairs. These large dark blotches indicate that her brain was working harder than it should have been to recall the words, yet her memory tests still showed an average score for her age group. So, like most people, she simply had normal aging.

Helen's anxiety about her memory slips motivated her to begin protecting her brain against Alzheimer's disease, so she closely followed the details of her Alzheimer's prevention program. She ate the right foods, worked out every day, made efforts to reduce her stress, and diligently practiced her memory exercises.

The MRI scan results of her brain stress test after about a week on the Alzheimer's prevention program showed much lower activity in her brain memory centers (meaning her brain wasn't struggling); however, her memory performance scores had improved dramatically. With minimal neural activation, her memory ability had increased more than 100 percent above her baseline levels. She now had the cognitive skills of a 35-year-old. One week on the Alzheimer's prevention program had subtracted 16 years from her brain age. Like many baby boomers, once Helen experienced the benefits of a healthy brain lifestyle, she was hooked. Helen had a reasonably healthy lifestyle before she started the Alzheimer's prevention program: She wasn't a smoker, only drank a glass of wine at dinner on weekends, and was not overweight. She was typical of many of our patients and research volunteers who begin healthy and yet still experience benefits in the first week.

Our other UCLA volunteers showed similar results—their brains got an efficiency jump-start, working more smoothly and easily, like a well-oiled machine that is less likely to break down. The Alzheimer's prevention program clearly

Q: **I know that severe head trauma can cause brain injury, but how bad does it have to be to increase your risk for Alzheimer's?**

A: Getting knocked out for an hour or more can double your risk for developing Alzheimer's disease; repeated minor concussions are bad for the brain, as well. Soccer players score lower than other athletes on memory tests, presumably due to repeated trauma from headers. Professional football players have higher rates of dementia at earlier ages in life. This doesn't mean that your soccer champion of a child will necessarily experience memory problems, but it does mean that it is important to try to protect our brains from possible head trauma—if you ride a bike, wear a helmet; and try to avoid sports that put your head at risk for concussion.

improved brain efficiency: the volunteers' brains could accomplish more while exerting less energy in the same way our bodies respond to a physical fitness program. The first few times you go to the gym and lift a 20-pound weight, you may get sore. But after a week or two of training, you not only don't get sore, you can probably lift heavier weight while your muscles exert less energy.

The sooner you start to protect your brain against Alzheimer's, the sooner you will notice improvement—not only in recall and mental focus, but also in energy level, mood, general health, and sense of well-being. And once you experience these results, you'll be hooked, too.

"SELF-KNOWLEDGE
IS THE BEGINNING OF
SELF-IMPROVEMENT."

—BALTASAR GRACIÁN,
17TH-CENTURY SPANISH WRITER

# Where You Stand Now

D R. HAROLD G., A 70-YEAR-OLD COLLEAGUE, was having trouble keeping track of appointments and remembering names. He was still active in his field of research, but his memory lapses worried him—they seemed to be getting worse every year. Harold knew about my Alzheimer's prevention research, but he figured he was too old to get much out of it. I insisted he was wrong. Unless you're already suffering from significant Alzheimer's disease, it's never too late to start protecting your brain. And if you are already experiencing some symptoms of dementia, this program can help you ward off further deterioration.

When I asked if he exercised, he said he used to play tennis with his wife, but since she passed away nine years ago, he really didn't get out much. He also didn't bother to cook meals very often and instead ate at fast-food restaurants. It was easy to recognize several lifestyle changes Harold could make to defend his brain against Alzheimer's.

I urged him to get a baseline assessment. He protested. I'm not sure he really wanted to know what was happening to his memory. However, with some prodding, he finally agreed to a standard assessment similar to the one that follows in this chapter. First he completed a questionnaire that rated his *subjective memory* (his own perception of his ability to remember), and then we assessed his *objective memory* (how he actually performed on a memory test). I also took into account his medical condition, physical fitness, diet, stress level, and other lifestyle habits that might affect his memory ability and his risk for Alzheimer's disease.

As Harold and I reviewed his results, I discussed his strengths and weaknesses and highlighted the lifestyle habits he could modify to protect his brain. When Harold saw his assessment scores in black and white, he finally made the connection between his everyday behaviors and his risk for Alzheimer's disease. That insight motivated him to start playing tennis again and even go back to the gym. He also began eating a healthier diet and doing mental exercises to sharpen his thinking. When he returned to my office four months later for a reassessment, his memory scores had improved by 30 percent.

Many people who complain or joke about their age-related memory changes start out like Harold, reluctant to get a baseline assessment. Some would rather stay in denial than really know if their memory is declining, even though that knowledge could give them a starting point for lowering their risk for Alzheimer's disease. But once people do know their baseline, they often see the correlation between their brain health and their daily behaviors, and that motivates them to adjust their lifestyle. Systematic studies have confirmed that this type of knowledge is a powerful incentive to engage in a healthy lifestyle.

This chapter offers some do-it-yourself assessment tools to help guide you on how to start protecting your brain and lowering your risk for Alzheimer's disease. The questionnaires and assessments are adapted from those I have used with thousands of patients and volunteers in my clinical practice and research studies. The measures are simple to use and can help you easily grasp where you stand in your brain's aging trajectory. The goal is to create a personalized Alzheimer's prevention program that meets your needs, builds on your strengths, and addresses any weaknesses.

## Memory Changes That You Notice

Memory complaints are so common that in our studies of brain aging and Alzheimer's risk, we have found that nearly everyone from age 40 and up notices some type of memory decline compared to when they were younger, and they generally agree that it gets slightly worse as years go by. Our UCLA brain scan studies have shown that memory self-assessment, or *subjective* memory scores, often correlate with activity levels in brain memory centers, as well as actual buildup of brain amyloid plaques and tau tangles. Your answers may be just a subjective impression, but these impressions often point to real changes in brain structure and function.

Take out a pencil and complete the following assessment to rate your subjective memory. For every item, circle the number from 1 to 5 that best describes the frequency (rarely, sometimes, or often) with which you experience each memory challenge. Then add up your subtotals for each area of memory ability, as well as your overall total at the bottom of the questionnaire. By using a pencil, you can erase your answers and return to these assessments later to gauge your improvement over time. You could also just use a different-colored pencil when you return to assess your progress.

# SUBJECTIVE MEMORY ASSESSMENT

| PEOPLE'S NAMES | RARELY | | SOMETIMES | | OFTEN |
|---|---|---|---|---|---|
| Recognizing a face but forgetting the person's name | 1 | 2 | 3 | 4 | 5 |
| Having to ask someone's name twice | 1 | 2 | 3 | 4 | 5 |
| Not being able to introduce someone when you see them out of context (e.g., running into a coworker at the movies) | 1 | 2 | 3 | 4 | 5 |
| Someone greets you using your name and you can't recall the person's name to greet them back | 1 | 2 | 3 | 4 | 5 |
| Scanning through the alphabet to try to remember someone's name | 1 | 2 | 3 | 4 | 5 |

TOTAL THE CIRCLED NUMBERS _____

| DIFFICULTY FINDING THINGS AND PLACES | RARELY | | SOMETIMES | | OFTEN |
|---|---|---|---|---|---|
| Objects you frequently use (glasses, keys, cell phone) | 1 | 2 | 3 | 4 | 5 |
| A parked car in a large lot | 1 | 2 | 3 | 4 | 5 |
| Receipts, tickets, documents | 1 | 2 | 3 | 4 | 5 |
| A store, business, or friend's home you've visited before | 1 | 2 | 3 | 4 | 5 |
| Things you rarely use (a book, file, etc.) | 1 | 2 | 3 | 4 | 5 |

TOTAL = _____

| TIP-OF-THE-TONGUE | RARELY | | SOMETIMES | | OFTEN |
|---|---|---|---|---|---|
| Trying to remember the title of a movie you just saw or a book you just read | 1 | 2 | 3 | 4 | 5 |
| Trouble finding the correct word for something | 1 | 2 | 3 | 4 | 5 |
| Knowing the answer to a question but it just won't come to mind | 1 | 2 | 3 | 4 | 5 |
| Not recalling what you wanted to say | 1 | 2 | 3 | 4 | 5 |
| Substituting an alternate word because you can't come up with the word you want | 1 | 2 | 3 | 4 | 5 |

TOTAL = _____

| EVENTS AND PLANS | RARELY | | SOMETIMES | | OFTEN |
|---|---|---|---|---|---|
| Forgetting an appointment or errand | 1 | 2 | 3 | 4 | 5 |
| Not remembering why you walked into a room | 1 | 2 | 3 | 4 | 5 |
| Forgetting to bring something important with you (e.g., a gift, file, etc.) | 1 | 2 | 3 | 4 | 5 |
| Coming home from the market without the original item you went for | 1 | 2 | 3 | 4 | 5 |
| Not remembering to call someone back | 1 | 2 | 3 | 4 | 5 |

TOTAL = _____

| ATTENTIVENESS | RARELY | | SOMETIMES | | OFTEN |
|---|---|---|---|---|---|
| Forgetting something someone just told you | 1 | 2 | 3 | 4 | 5 |
| Having to reread a paragraph you already read | 1 | 2 | 3 | 4 | 5 |
| Trouble following instructions or directions | 1 | 2 | 3 | 4 | 5 |
| Having to ask a question multiple times | 1 | 2 | 3 | 4 | 5 |
| Forgetting whether you already told somebody something | 1 | 2 | 3 | 4 | 5 |

TOTAL = _____

## ADD THE TOTALS TOGETHER FOR SUBJECTIVE MEMORY SCORE

Your subjective memory scores will guide you on how best to maintain and improve your current memory abilities. Your score for each category (for example, people's names, finding things and places) will give you a sense of specific memory areas you might want to improve. If you scored a total of 10 or less in any one of the categories, then you probably don't need to spend much time on that particular area. In fact, if you scored that well, many other baby boomers will want to know what you are doing to keep your memory in such great shape, so beware if you brag about your scores too much. If your score totaled 15 or more in any one area, you might consider spending more time practicing the exercises and techniques that will improve your skills in that area of memory performance.

Your overall score will give you a sense of your general subjective memory ability as of today. If your total score is 40 or less, your memory complaints are most likely minimal; however, learning new memory techniques will still help you strengthen your memory skills for the future. If your total score exceeds 70, you are probably experiencing the more frequent memory challenges that many people notice as they age. I suggest that you take extra time when learning new memory methods.

Even if your total score is high, there is no need to panic—plaques and tangles have not necessarily taken over your brain. It takes a long time for these tiny proteins to build up in our brains and cause any damage. Neurons can be resilient and return to normal function with practice. Our UCLA functional MRI scan studies have shown that

Q: **My grandmother and her sister both got Alzheimer's disease in their late 60s. I'm 45 now and wonder if I should get checked out.**

A: In less than 5 percent of families with Alzheimer's, half the relatives develop the disease early in life, usually before age 60. In these situations, family members are inheriting a gene that causes the disease, and genetic testing can inform them of whether they are carriers of the genetic mutation. Occasionally these autosomal dominant families (named for the pattern of inheritance) have a later onset of the disease. A genetic counselor can help you determine whether your family has this kind of inheritance pattern, and review the psychological impact of genetic testing.

even older, forgetful brains have the elasticity to bounce back to where they should be. Our brain exercise programs, whether they involve learning new memory techniques or simply to search online using a computer for the first time, lead to rapid and significant improvements in brain activity levels and higher memory performance scores within a week or two. If you don't find the exercises helpful and remain concerned about your scores, consider discussing your concerns with your physician.

## Objective Recall

Although subjective impressions of memory ability are important, by definition they are subjective, so we need to balance them with objective measures: those that can be backed up with solid data. One of the most useful objective memory measures is called *delayed recall.* It involves learning a list of unrelated words and then, after a 10-minute delay, recalling as many of the words as possible. Used extensively by neuropsychologists, this method is much more sensitive to subtle and early signs of brain aging than many other standardized mental assessments.

To determine your objective recall score, set a timer or stop watch for 1 minute. In that minute, memorize the word list on the following page. Ready, set, go.

After the minute, put down your book and reset the timer for 10 minutes. Distract yourself from the word list by doing something else: Clean out a drawer, read a magazine, or juggle some oranges, which by the way, will give your right brain hemisphere a workout. The point is to take your mind off the list so that the delayed recall assessment is accurate. When your timer alerts you in 10 minutes, get a pen and paper and write down as many of the words as you can recall without looking back at the list.

This kind of assessment is helpful in detecting and tracking any subtle early signs of brain aging beyond the subjective memory measure.

# OBJECTIVE RECALL ASSESSMENT

**tuna**

**parachute**

**truck**

**valley**

**telephone**

**climber**

**lizard**

**cave**

**tea bag**

**bowl**

RECORD YOUR OBJECTIVE RECALL
SCORE HERE

Your score is the total number of correct words you can write down after the 10-minute break. You need to write the exact word, so if you write down fish instead of tuna, you miss a point. Record your score.

Your objective recall score may be consistent with the results of your subjective memory score. In other words, the memory challenges you are noticing are actually present when you test for them objectively. Sometimes, however, the memory self-assessment score indicates more difficulties than indicated on the objective recall score. That kind of mismatch often points to anxiety and stress, suggesting that the individual is overly worried about every middle-age pause or senior moment, perhaps perceiving them as signals that rapid mental decline or impending Alzheimer's disease is just around the corner. If your objective recall score is 5 or more and your subjective memory score indicates that you are often noticing memory changes (total score is greater than 70), your baseline memory performance is pretty good and you probably worry too much about your memory. Worrying about memory problems only makes memory performance worse. I advise people who are anxious about their memory challenges to focus on stress management when they individualize their Alzheimer's prevention programs.

## Physical Fitness

In recent years, compelling scientific evidence has shown that staying physically fit is a key component of defending against Alzheimer's disease. Studies show that aerobic training improves brain function as we age, especially in the neural circuits that control memory, reasoning, and attention.

To get an idea of your current level of physical conditioning, complete the following rating scale to assess each of these three major areas: (1) aerobic conditioning, (2) strength training, and (3) balance and stability. Circle the number between 1 and 5 that best describes your current physical abilities.

# PHYSICAL FITNESS QUESTIONNAIRE

| AEROBIC CONDITIONING | RARELY | | SOMETIMES | | OFTEN |
|---|---|---|---|---|---|
| Getting winded from climbing two flights of stairs | 1 | 2 | 3 | 4 | 5 |
| Feeling fatigued or out of breath from taking a brisk walk | 1 | 2 | 3 | 4 | 5 |
| Choosing the elevator over the stairs | 1 | 2 | 3 | 4 | 5 |
| Preferring to drive a few blocks rather than walking | 1 | 2 | 3 | 4 | 5 |
| Making excuses to avoid physical exertion | 1 | 2 | 3 | 4 | 5 |

**TOTAL THE CIRCLED NUMBERS** _____

| STRENGTH TRAINING | RARELY | | SOMETIMES | | OFTEN |
|---|---|---|---|---|---|
| Difficulty lifting heavy objects | 1 | 2 | 3 | 4 | 5 |
| Concerned about shaking hands with someone who might have a firm grip | 1 | 2 | 3 | 4 | 5 |
| Unable to stand unsupported (e.g., waiting in line) for 15 minutes or longer | 1 | 2 | 3 | 4 | 5 |
| Difficulty opening a window or twisting open a jar top | 1 | 2 | 3 | 4 | 5 |
| Asking others to lift or carry things for you | 1 | 2 | 3 | 4 | 5 |

**TOTAL =** _____

| BALANCE AND STABILITY | RARELY | | SOMETIMES | | OFTEN |
|---|---|---|---|---|---|
| Losing balance while standing up or sitting down | 1 | 2 | 3 | 4 | 5 |
| Fear of tripping or falling while walking | 1 | 2 | 3 | 4 | 5 |
| Inability to stand on one leg for more than 5 seconds | 1 | 2 | 3 | 4 | 5 |
| Having to sit to put on loafers or slip on shoes | 1 | 2 | 3 | 4 | 5 |
| Feeling unsteady or needing to use a handrail when walking up or down stairs | 1 | 2 | 3 | 4 | 5 |

**TOTAL =** _____

---

ADD THE TOTALS TOGETHER FOR
PHYSICAL FITNESS SCORE

---

If you score a total of 10 or less in any category, you are in pretty good physical shape, and your Alzheimer's prevention program will help you further improve your physical health. If you scored 15 or more in any one category, you should spend extra time on exercises to improve your fitness in that area. In addition, your overall score provides you with a measure of your general fitness. If your total score is 30 or less, you are in pretty good shape; but if your total score exceeds 35, improving your physical fitness is likely to have an impact on your brain fitness.

Optimizing physical health requires attention to medical issues, especially for middle-aged and older individuals who typically suffer from multiple medical ailments. Staying physically healthy can help prevent and manage chronic medical conditions such as diabetes and high blood pressure. People with arthritis sometimes need to adjust their fitness routines to accommodate physical limitations, so swimming may be a safer option than jogging.

# Dietary Habits

In my research and clinical practice, I find that of all the lifestyle habits I recommend, people seem most resistant to changing their diet, yet that is one of the first areas where they notice the most compelling benefits. An Alzheimer's prevention diet not only involves settling at the correct weight for your body type, but also eating the right kinds of fats, proteins, and carbohydrates. To get a sense of how healthy your current eating habits are, circle the numbers on the next page that indicate your strengths and weaknesses:

# HEALTHY BRAIN
## DIET QUESTIONNAIRE

| CALORIE INTAKE | RARELY | | SOMETIMES | | OFTEN |
|---|---|---|---|---|---|
| Feeling too full after eating a meal | 1 | 2 | 3 | 4 | 5 |
| Drinking sodas or sugared beverages | 1 | 2 | 3 | 4 | 5 |
| Worrying about your body weight | 1 | 2 | 3 | 4 | 5 |
| Having to buy bigger clothes | 1 | 2 | 3 | 4 | 5 |
| Noticing that your stomach is larger than it used to be | 1 | 2 | 3 | 4 | 5 |

TOTAL THE CIRCLED NUMBERS _____

| FATS AND PROTEINS | RARELY | | SOMETIMES | | OFTEN |
|---|---|---|---|---|---|
| Choosing steaks or burgers for entrées | 1 | 2 | 3 | 4 | 5 |
| Eating fried foods | 1 | 2 | 3 | 4 | 5 |
| Opting for ice cream or a fatty dessert | 1 | 2 | 3 | 4 | 5 |
| Avoiding fish and lean chicken | 1 | 2 | 3 | 4 | 5 |
| Using butter on bread or popcorn | 1 | 2 | 3 | 4 | 5 |

TOTAL = _____

| CARBOHYDRATES | RARELY | | SOMETIMES | | OFTEN |
|---|---|---|---|---|---|
| Snacking on candy or cookies | 1 | 2 | 3 | 4 | 5 |
| Eating white bread or dinner rolls | 1 | 2 | 3 | 4 | 5 |
| Having donuts, pancakes, or waffles for breakfast | 1 | 2 | 3 | 4 | 5 |
| Choosing processed foods (e.g., pasta) over whole whole grains (e.g., quinoa or barley) | 1 | 2 | 3 | 4 | 5 |
| Having trouble stopping yourself from finishing the whole bag of whatever you're eating | 1 | 2 | 3 | 4 | 5 |

TOTAL = _____

## TOTAL HEALTHY BRAIN DIET SCORE

Total your scores in each of the three areas at left to help you get started on an Alzheimer's prevention nutrition plan. If you score 10 or less in any of the areas, then your current nutritional habits are likely protecting your body and your brain. An overall score of 30 or less indicates that your diet is fairly healthy; however, scores greater than 35 indicate that you should pay more attention to your nutritional choices in your Alzheimer's prevention program.

One of the most common challenges is calorie intake and weight control. As people age, they tend to gain weight.

The National Institutes of Health have provided a formula to help people calculate their ideal body weight. For men, the NIH recommends calculating 106 pounds for the first five feet of height and adding 6 pounds to the total weight for every inch above five feet. So for a man who is 5 feet 9 inches tall, his ideal body weight would be 106 pounds plus 54 pounds (i.e., 6 pounds times 9) or 160 pounds. For women, NIH suggests starting with 100 pounds of body weight for the first 5 feet of height and then adding 5 pounds for each additional inch. Using this formula, a woman who is 5 feet 4 inches would have an ideal body weight of 120 pounds (100 plus 20 pounds). Now, use these formulas to calculate your ideal body weight. Write it down in the space below, and then write down your actual body weight for comparison.

---

### YOUR CALCULATED IDEAL BODY WEIGHT

### YOUR BASELINE BODY WEIGHT

# STRESS LEVEL ASSESSMENT SCALE

| PSYCHOLOGICAL SYMPTOMS | RARELY | | SOMETIMES | | OFTEN |
|---|---|---|---|---|---|
| Worrying about things that aren't even important the next day | 1 | 2 | 3 | 4 | 5 |
| Anticipating the worst | 1 | 2 | 3 | 4 | 5 |
| Feeling tense, irritable, or impatient | 1 | 2 | 3 | 4 | 5 |
| Unable to stop ruminating about things that are bothering you | 1 | 2 | 3 | 4 | 5 |
| A sense of hopelessness that things will ever get better | 1 | 2 | 3 | 4 | 5 |

TOTAL THE CIRCLED NUMBERS _____

| PHYSICAL SYMPTOMS | RARELY | | SOMETIMES | | OFTEN |
|---|---|---|---|---|---|
| Trouble falling asleep, waking throughout the night, or daytime fatigue | 1 | 2 | 3 | 4 | 5 |
| Nervous twitches, fidgeting, or restlessness | 1 | 2 | 3 | 4 | 5 |
| Rapid heart rate, dry mouth, or shortness of breath | 1 | 2 | 3 | 4 | 5 |
| Decreased or increased appetite | 1 | 2 | 3 | 4 | 5 |
| Headaches, neck pain, or upset stomach | 1 | 2 | 3 | 4 | 5 |

TOTAL = _____

| COPING ABILITIES | RARELY | | SOMETIMES | | OFTEN |
|---|---|---|---|---|---|
| Failing to follow through on things | 1 | 2 | 3 | 4 | 5 |
| Avoiding strategies to reduce stress (meditation, physical exercise, etc.) | 1 | 2 | 3 | 4 | 5 |
| Indecisiveness | 1 | 2 | 3 | 4 | 5 |
| Inability to hide your anxiety from others | 1 | 2 | 3 | 4 | 5 |
| Difficulty seeking help | 1 | 2 | 3 | 4 | 5 |

TOTAL = _____

## ADD THE TOTALS TOGETHER FOR STRESS LEVEL SCORE

## Stress Levels

Everyone suffers from stress at certain points in their life, and many of us face a daily onslaught of worries, demands, and uncertainties that take their toll on our brain health. Chronic stress not only diminishes our quality of life, but it increases our risk for developing Alzheimer's disease. Although we cannot eliminate all external causes of stress, we can learn to manage our stress triggers better and lower their impact on our neuronal stability.

People's ability to cope with stress differs. The chart on the facing page will give you a better sense of how much stress disrupts your life.

Your scores in each of the categories at left give you an estimate of your current level of stress. If your score totals 10 or less in any of the areas, then you either live a very serene lifestyle or you've figured out a way to cope with everyday stressors. A score of 15 or more in any one category indicates you may want to focus on reducing your stress in that area. Your overall score will help gauge how much attention you need to pay on stress reduction in general. If your total overall score is greater than 35, then stress management should be a priority in your Alzheimer's prevention program.

## Keep Track of Your Progress

By completing your baseline assessments, you have taken the first step to protecting your brain from Alzheimer's disease. You can use the charts in Appendix 1, as well as the questionnaires here, to enter your baseline scores and later reassess your abilities and gauge your progress. Stay on your new program and you are sure to see steady improvement.

"MY DOCTOR SAYS TOO
MUCH SEX CAN CAUSE
MEMORY LOSS.
NOW, WHAT WAS I
ABOUT TO SAY?"

—MILTON BERLE

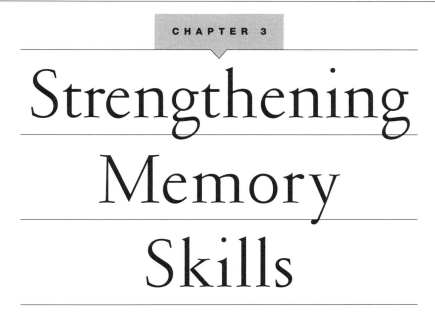

# Strengthening Memory Skills

J EFF C. WAS A BIT NERVOUS ABOUT ATTENDING
PARENTS' NIGHT at his daughter's school without
his wife. She always knew everybody and prompted
him on people's names if he forgot them. He slipped in
quietly; luckily for Jeff, he was pretty sure he knew the
name of the first person he spotted across the room. As he
walked up to him, he ran the alphabet through his head—
just in case—and stopped at *K*. "Ken, it's great to see you
again. Can you believe these kids are seniors already?"

Ken shook his head and said, "It's amazing, Jeff. Where
does the time go?"

Jeff was relieved. He had gotten the guy's name right. As he glanced around for other people he might know, he felt that tonight might not be as bad as he thought. With renewed confidence, Jeff said, "So how's work, Ken? And is your lovely wife here with you tonight?" Jeff couldn't remember her name and was hoping that Ken would say it.

"Barbara's meeting me here after work," Ken said. "She'll be here any minute."

Jeff started thinking . . . Barbara, Barbara, got to remember Ken and Barbara, just like Ken and Barbie, but not the doll. Barbara.

Ken interrupted Jeff's ruminations. "You all right Jeff? Want a drink or something?"

"No, thanks, Ken, I'm good."

A couple approached them, and the man said to Ken, "Kevin, you dog. Where have you been hiding?"

Jeff swallowed hard and suddenly noticed that Ken was wearing a name tag on his lapel that clearly read "Hi. I'm Kevin."

Jeff's episode of mistaken identity could happen to anyone. He was struggling to come up with a way to jog his memory, but his alphabet association was doomed from the beginning, since he missed the obvious name tag. Remember, if you're not sure about somebody's name and he happens to be wearing a name tag, check it out.

In everyday life, people don't usually wear name tags, so we need other methods to help us overcome one of the most common forms of age-related memory decline: recalling names. Sometimes the same memory strategy that helps us remember names can help us deal with other common memory challenges, including misplacing things, recalling words we want to say, and remembering plans and appointments.

This chapter will review several memory enhancement strategies to help us choose the right one for any situation. With practice, these methods will build your confidence, which can further strengthen your memory ability. Because memory decline is one of the earliest symptoms of Alzheimer's disease, keeping our memory abilities sharp is an essential part of any Alzheimer's prevention program.

## What Is Memory?

Memory defines who we are. Without our memories we have no past, cannot plan for the future, and have no context for appreciating the present.

Memory consists of two major components: getting information into our brains (learning) and retrieving that information later (recall). Forming new memories and recalling them later involves a complex array of biochemical events, electrical transmissions, and neuronal connections that occur throughout the brain.

From moment to moment, our brains are bombarded with numerous external and internal stimuli. We observe, hear, smell, taste, and feel a multitude of stimuli from the outside environment; at the same time, we're responding to internal cues—various thoughts, emotions, and sensations. Our nervous systems create a very brief record of all this information as we experience it. This brief record is called *sensory memory*. A sensory memory could be seeing a traffic light turn to green or feeling the shower water as too hot.

Q: I am 50 and my memory is worse than when I was 20. Could this be Alzheimer's disease?

A: Probably not. Memory changes are normal as we get older. The risk for Alzheimer's is less than 1% at age 50.

If the brain continuously focused on all its incoming stimuli, it would be overwhelmed like a computer that has maxed out its RAM. To function in the world, we can't possibly remember every bit of sensory input. Our brains instinctively pluck out the important information and retain it in *short-term memory*. This short-term memory, also known as *working memory*, allows us to carry out quick tasks, like responding to an e-mail or hearing a phone number from directory assistance and remembering it just long enough to dial it. Working memory stores information for a very brief period, a bit like disappearing ink on a note pad.

If we want to retain information for more than just a few moments, our brains have to push it through to *long-term memory*. Only a few sensory memories make it to short-term memory, and even fewer short-term memories become stored as long-term ones, as illustrated below.

| SENSORY MEMORIES | SHORT-TERM MEMORIES | LONG-TERM MEMORIES |
| --- | --- | --- |
| dog barking | | |
| towel on floor | | |
| name of waiter ⟶ | name of waiter | |
| scald from hot water ⟶ | scald from hot water ⟶ | scald from hot water |
| sex on honeymoon ⟶ | sex on honeymoon ⟶ | sex on honeymoon |
| hot car seat ⟶ | hot car seat | |
| phone ringing | | |
| smog in the morning | | |
| smell of roses in garden | | |

The process involves filtering out extraneous details and honing in on the important elements of the experience or information we wish to remember. This data storage procedure involves organizing the information so that it has meaning and often relates to other, already-stored memories. Your recollection of your first car at age 16 is probably linked to an emotional memory of feeling independent and free. Perhaps even to making out in the backseat. If you remember back to your first apartment, you may smile when you recall the milk crates you used for bookshelves.

During this storage process, the brain changes itself in order to solidify these permanent memories. Brain cells extend their axons, the long "wires" connecting them to other cells, and the connection sites, or synapses, between the cells become more efficient at releasing the chemical messages needed for memory storage and retrieval. For one memory to enter the brain requires several parts of the brain to work together.

# Memory Neighborhoods

I was driving with Gigi, trying to remember who had told me a joke a few weeks earlier. As I came to a stop sign, I saw a coffee shop and blurted out, "Don Siegel!"

Gigi looked at me as if I were insane. "What about him?"

"There . . . at Starbucks," I said. "That's where he told me the joke."

"What joke?" she asked, shaking her head.

Just as my memory was jogged by the neighborhood where I was driving, our memories live in neighborhoods, or particular regions in our brains. Jog a part of a memory in one section of the brain and the neural connections will signal the cells in another part of the memory neighborhood to pull together the information you're trying to recall. Part of a memory neighborhood may be physically right next door to another section of the brain; another part may be on the opposite side, with long axons connecting the two.

**TRY THIS!**

To cross-train your brain, brush your teeth with your opposite hand. Don't forget to floss.

Sometimes these memory neighborhoods get too crowded with memories, forcing us to move some of our memories out to the suburbs. Neuroscientists at Yale University found that when the brain is cluttered with similar memories, the memories compete, making recall of the correct one more difficult. This memory retrieval competition results in less focused and more ambiguous patterns of brain activation. The brain may retrieve the wrong competing memory and show weaker activation of regions associated with the target memory. For instance, we could mix up the lyrics of a song on the oldies station while singing along. The good news is that we can learn simple memory techniques to help us focus on the memories we want to retrieve and avoid the distraction of competing memories.

One way the brain avoids these kinds of distraction is through its inborn organizational structure based on different functional regions. If, perhaps, you were at a rock concert, you would be hearing the music,

49

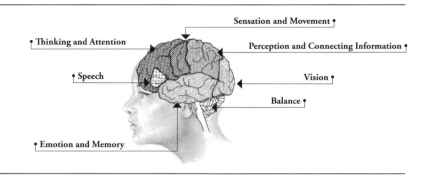

Thinking and Attention

Speech

Emotion and Memory

Sensation and Movement

Perception and Connecting Information

Vision

Balance

seeing the performers, feeling the urge to dance, and possibly even smelling a nontobacco smoke odor. Your brain would process each of these sensations and record them in separate regions, creating a unique memory neighborhood for this particular event. You might also be thinking about how much older the musicians look since the last time you saw them perform. Or perhaps you might notice how much older the audience looks than the last time—except for yourself, of course. To consolidate this rock-concert memory neighborhood, your neural axons would be connecting regions throughout the brain that control hearing, vision, smell, and thought, as well as any other areas that are possibly being stimulated by talking to your friend, dancing, or drinking a soda. One brain area that is particularly powerful in linking an event to long-term memory is the temporal lobe, located under the temples. This area processes emotions.

## Emotional Memory

I can vividly recall the first time I met Gigi, our wedding day, the birth of our first child, Rachel, and the day Rachel uttered her first word: *Agua* ("water" in Spanish). Gigi was thrilled that her precious one-year-old had talked, but realized that she had better stop working so much and give the babysitter more days off.

Most of us remember what we were doing when we heard about

the Kennedy assassinations or the 9/11 disaster, but we probably have little or no recall of the week leading up to those events. Emotional memories can be positive, negative, or both, but either way, they tend to go straight into long-term memory stores and stay there. We're also much more likely to remember an exciting experience than a boring one. Memory enhancement techniques are generally more effective when we charge them with an emotional component, although sometimes too much emotion can distract us and distort our memories.

Within the temporal lobe, these emotional memories are processed by the amygdala (*uh-mig-del-uh*), which sits right next to the hippocampus, a horseshoe-shaped brain region that is essential for forming new memories. Damage to the hippocampus can cause several forms of amnesia, including anterograde (inability to create new memories) and retrograde (inability to remember anything before the damage occurred).

The hippocampus and the amygdala are also neighbors of the olfactory bulb, the brain region that controls our sense of smell. There are many nerve connections between these regions, which may explain why odors can be such powerful emotional memory triggers.

## Memory and the Aging Brain

As we get older, almost all of us notice a decline in our memory abilities. Most of us are able to cope with occasional memory slips and even joke about them. When scientists study the effects of aging on memory, they find that an older brain often needs more time to process new information. This slower processing speed affects all forms of memory: sensory, short-term, and long-term.

Although an older brain is more susceptible to memory lapses and pathology that can lead to Alzheimer's disease, the middle-aged brain (age 35 to 55) has a sweet spot when it becomes especially agile. During this period, the brain becomes more efficient at processing available information it has gathered over its lifetime. Vocabulary has been shown to improve during middle age, and neuroscientists believe that a growth spurt of the brain's white matter may explain its neural agility. UCLA scientists have found significantly higher quantities of white matter coating the axonal wires of the neurons in middle-aged brains. This white matter serves as insulation for the long axons and facilitates more efficient communication between cells, allowing them to transmit information at an accelerated rate. While middle-agers complain about forgetting where they put their keys or glasses, many also notice their improved skills at running a business, seeing the big picture of things, and figuring out novel ways to solve their short-term memory issues.

Q: I have always had a bad memory. Will a memory course help me now that I'm already in my 60s, or is it a waste of time?

A: Although most people take memory classes because they have noticed worsening of their memory abilities as they age, the methods taught can help people with memory challenges due to a variety of causes. Simple techniques, such as *LOOK, SNAP, CONNECT* and the story method (see pp. 54 and 55), have been found to improve memory performance regardless of how long someone has experienced memory challenges.

The independent right and left hemispheres of the brain also begin to communicate better as the brain ages. In children, adolescents, and young adults, these two sides of the brain work more independently—one side may be listening to music while the other side searches online. Studies have shown that older individuals demonstrate improved mental abilities when both sides of their brains work on a task together. In people with mild cognitive impairment, memory training not only improves cognitive performance, but it engages a large network of brain regions that start working together during learning and recall. Our brains can remain malleable even as plaques and tangles build up in sensitive memory centers.

Wear and tear over the years does take its toll on neurons, but our brains naturally compensate when neurons misfire. My UCLA research indicates that the memory abilities of people who have a genetic risk for Alzheimer's disease are as good as those of people without the genetic risk, but their brains may have to work harder to perform a memory task in order to compensate for subtle age-related declines.

Unfortunately for many people, their compensation strategies ultimately break down and they eventually show some symptoms of Alzheimer's disease. Regardless of whether or not someone has a genetic risk for Alzheimer's, if they decide to take charge of their brain health, they may be able to stave off some Alzheimer's symptoms for years by learning and practicing memory enhancement techniques.

# Memory Training 101

Scientific evidence shows that practicing basic memory methods sharpens memory capacity, slows age-related decline, and helps maintain peak memory performance. If we use these methods regularly, we can enjoy better memory skills and sustain them for years.

Our UCLA research group has found that using simple memory techniques can activate and strengthen specific neural circuits in the brain's frontal lobe, a critically important memory-processing center. As we learn memory enhancement skills, neural activity increases as the brain recruits neighboring circuits to solve tasks. With practice, the brain develops more efficient strategies for both learning and recall and eventually neural activity decreases as the brain uses less energy to do the same tasks. This is why an effective prevention strategy provides several levels of brain exercises so we can continually stimulate the brain with more and more challenging exercises as it becomes more efficient.

These methods do more than just tweak our axons and *dendrites*, the short nerve cell extensions that receive messages from other cells. They have a real impact on memory performance. For example, a ten-session memory training course was found to improve everyday functioning and cognitive abilities in nearly 3,000 older adults (age 65 and up), and those benefits were still observed five years after the intervention.

Systematic studies also show that we can train the brain to perform specific mental skills, ranging from calculation ability to verbal reasoning. Unless you have a yearning to become a mathematical wizard or you are particularly keen on being a contestant on *Jeopardy!*, you are probably just looking to improve your memory performance in the areas where most people first notice decline as they age:

- *names and faces*
- *where we put things*
- *what we plan to do*
- *tip-of-the-tongue phenomena*

In addition to describing how my basic memory strategy *LOOK, SNAP, CONNECT* can be used to improve learning and recall and help us overcome the most annoying memory challenges, I will introduce exercises that target these and other common problems.

## Look, Snap, Connect

When Gigi and I were first writing about memory, we were trying to come up with a short-hand term for the basic components of nearly all memory techniques: focusing attention, creating visual images, and linking these images together. I pitched her something I called my three P's: *P*ay attention, *P*rint a mental photograph, and *P*ut those photographs together in a bundle.

She laughed, "The three *P*'s? Like the three little pigs or do they come in a pod?"

"Hey, I'm trying here."

"How about something like Look, Snap, Connect?" she asked.

"That's exactly what I meant."

- *LOOK*: Focus your attention on what you want to recall later. When we're distracted, we don't fully take note of the information.

- *SNAP*: Form a visual image or mental snapshot of the information you want to learn. Our brains have evolved to remember images best, so they've become hard-wired to recall visual information.

- *CONNECT*: Create visual associations to connect up your mental snapshots for later recall. This step links the new information to make it meaningful and easy to retrieve later.

*LOOK, SNAP,* and *CONNECT* are the three basic skills that can help us remember people's names, appointments, lists, where we put things, or just about any common memory task.

Try this method out by learning some unrelated word pairs. The memory challenge is to be able to associate two words so you can recall the second word after seeing the first one.

To begin, focus your attention (*LOOK*) on the following word pairs:

**rabbit — telephone**
**policeman — apple**

Next imagine a picture (*SNAP*) for each word and link the snaps (*CONNECT*) into one new image, like a rabbit talking on a telephone or a policeman eating an apple. The associations can be logical or illogical. In fact, sometimes the more unusual or bizarre the connection, the easier it is to recall later. Now you try the next two:

**keys — chopstick**
**rooster — hammock**

Did you imagine a snapshot of your keys dangling from a chopstick? Or perhaps a rooster relaxing on a hammock? If you did, you're on the right track, although there are many other possible snaps you may have imagined, such as forgetting your keys in a Chinese restaurant or a rooster awakening someone from a nap on a hammock.

You can build on the word pair exercise to apply it to a longer list of words and create a story that connects several snaps you've imagined. To practice this *story method*, focus on each word below and create a mental snap for each one. Next try to create a story that connects them. The order of the words can vary depending on your story line, and you can recall them in any order that works for you.

nun
bench
cigar
kite
lawyer
teddy bear

Now that you've created a story of your own, here's an example of one volunteer's narrative: A *nun* is sitting on a *bench*, smoking a *cigar* and flying a *kite*. A *lawyer* carrying a *teddy bear* sits down next to her and introduces himself and his bear.

Your story may be completely different. The lawyer may be smoking the cigar and flying the kite, or perhaps the teddy bear is fond of cigars and kites. Hey, the nun might even be a lawyer. Either way, giving the snaps meaning is the key to remembering the words.

You'll notice that the volunteer's story had interaction, silliness, and plenty of detail. The way mental snaps connect tends to be more memorable when we add detail and action, and even make it playful. Also, our first association to an image is often the easiest to recall later.

Now try the following exercises to fine-tune your mental snapshot skills:

1. For each of the following words, imagine a detailed, active mental snap (e.g., instead of a two-dimensional drawing of a dog, see a white, manicured poodle drinking from a water bowl).

dog
tree
river
desk

2. To build your imaginative abilities, try to visualize an outlandish snap for each of the following words (e.g., for "car," rather than picturing a black Prius parked in your

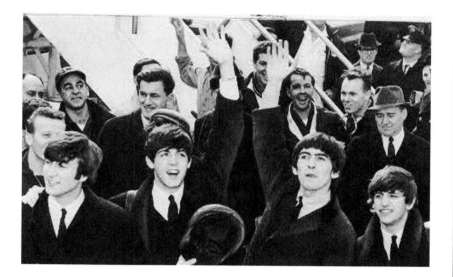

driveway, see a pink Mercedes with wings flying across the skyline).

car

**hammer**

park

**banana**

**3.** Look at this old photograph of the Beatles. Spend 30 seconds studying the photo; then put aside the book and write down as many details as you can recall.

How did you do? Did you remember which Beatles have their hands in the air? Whose arm is on John's shoulder? Are they wearing ties? Did you notice any policemen in the photo? How many? Did it seem like a warm or cold day? Why? Was anyone wearing glasses?

With practice, you'll find that your observation skills will sharpen and your mind will automatically create shortcuts for snaps and connects, much like a computer uses macros or programs to complete a word or correct your spelling. Also, keep in mind that emotional memories are often the most powerful and that our first associations with a snap or connections of snaps can be the most effective. Even though visual images seem to work best for most of us, *LOOK* can be a reminder to focus and pay attention to all five of your senses: seeing, hearing, feeling, smelling, and tasting.

Learning unrelated word pairs and word lists can help us build our basic memory skills, and we can easily transfer these skills to overcome common memory challenges. Let's say I need to run to the market, but I don't have a pad and pencil to jot down a shopping list. I can use *LOOK, SNAP, CONNECT* along with *chunking* to quickly remember the items I need. Chunking is a strategy that simply groups similar items into chunks or categories.

Rather than remembering six or more unrelated items to buy at the store, I chunk my grocery items into three categories depending on where I store them: the pantry, refrigerator, or freezer. That way, I need to remember only two or three short stories or word pairs. I look in my pantry for what I might need and create a mental snap of granola cereal pouring out of a can of tomato soup. Then I move on to the refrigerator, where I picture a quart of milk surrounded by a dozen oranges. Finally, I check the freezer and visualize a snap of a frozen chicken holding a pint of frozen vanilla yogurt. My shopping spree is a big success, although I did forget to buy a pad and pencil for future market lists.

## Never Forget What's-Her-Name

I'm walking down the street and I see someone familiar approaching in the distance. As she gets closer, I recognize the face—someone I knew several years ago, maybe before I was even married. Was it in L.A.? Boston? Did we work together? Date? I mentally search my rusty brain cells for the name . . . I know I'm going to come up with it . . . I just need a little more time, so I slow my gait a bit, but what's-her-name is coming toward me at a rapid clip. It's too late; I'm caught. I can't even duck behind a trash bin.

She smiles and says, "Hey, Gary, good to see you."

Of course, she remembers me perfectly *and* uses my name. Embarrassed, I stop and say, "It's great to see *you*." After a couple minutes of chitchat, I realize I'm behind schedule and tell her, "I've got to run, I'm late. All the best to the family." Once she's out of sight, I suddenly remember that *Carol* was a resident who supervised me when I was in medical school.

It's impossible to remember the name of everyone we've ever met, but with practice we can avoid many embarrassing situations by improving our ability to connect names to faces and recall them at will. The strategy is to use *LOOK, SNAP, CONNECT:* create a *name snap* and a *face snap*, and then connect them. I might picture Carol in a doctor's white coat, back in medical school, singing a Christmas carol. Of course, we can't always prepare in advance to avoid all name lapses, but I probably won't forget Carol's name again, although I may not see her for another ten years. Even if it's too late to use the Dr.-Carol-singing technique on her now, practicing it will keep it from happening in the future and my brain will become a bit stronger thanks to that practice.

While name snaps give us visual images to recall names (sometimes with an audio component such as the Christmas carol), face snaps help us associate a distinguishing facial feature or personal trait of the person we want to remember. For some names and faces it comes easy. Perhaps Mrs. Glass wears silly glasses or Mr. Sanders has sandy-colored hair. The connection doesn't have to be perfect—just close enough to jog your memory.

Some names readily evoke a visual image, like Bill (dollar bill), Cliff (precipice), Iris (flower), or Taylor (seamstress). Sometimes we have to use our imagination a bit when we meet a Philip (screwdriver) or a Haley (comet). I also find it helpful to associate faces with famous people from the past (when I meet Dr. Jefferson, I can easily visualize shaking hands with a founding father) or celebrities (when I meet Mr. Roberts, I imagine him hugging Julia Roberts—lucky guy).

For more complex names, I sometimes spell out the name in my mind's eye in order to visualize it, or I break it down into syllables that lend themselves to more memorable and connectable snaps. If I meet Jim Agronsky, I picture him lifting weights in a gym (Jim), a-groaning (Agron-) and wearing ski clothes (-sky).

See what images you can create for the following names:

**Joan Krebs**

**Hans Rosenwald**

**Aria Gilchrest**

I'm sure your snaps will be different from mine, but for Joan Krebs, I pictured Joan of Arc eating a crab salad. For Hans Rosenwald, I imagined his large hands tossing rose pedals against a wall. My Aria Gilchrest snap had her singing an operatic song while clutching a gull to her chest.

One reason we sometimes forget people's names right after we've been introduced is that we're not really paying full attention when we hear the name. Focusing attention is an important first step to learning new names and faces. Sometimes repeating a name and giving it personal meaning can help glue it to your memory stores. Also, when you meet someone for the first time, try to repeat their name during the conversation and use it when you say good-bye. If possible, share any associations you might have to the name during the conversation: "I have a cousin named Ellen. You remind me of her." You can also try to learn something about the person's life that interests you to help you remember the name later: "Your first name is Sigmund and you were born in Vienna? That's interesting."

Some of these techniques may feel odd at first, but the methods do work. My team at UCLA has trained thousands of people in these techniques, and our trainees have reported significantly better memory skills that many of them have sustained for years.

## Memory Places

I admit it. Years ago I misplaced my keys twice in one week. Gigi cured me of what she called my bad habit. She installed a series of hooks in our kitchen where all family members were to hang their keys.

Misplacing frequently used objects is one of the most common and easily correctable memory complaints that people report as they age. Gigi's simple strategy was to create a *memory place*. Park your car in the same general area every day at work. Put your keys, sunglasses, wallet, and cell phone in the same memory places every evening. Keep a pad and pen by the phone for messages. You may wish to put your calendar of upcoming appointments and events prominently on your desk or post it on a bulletin board. Be sure your memory places are logical and convenient.

When you're traveling, memory places can be more challenging. I usually designate one bedside or desk drawer in my hotel room for all my gadgets and documents: cell phone, laptop, wallet, keys, watch, receipts, itinerary, and anything else of importance. Of course, the large, framed picture of Gigi (I don't leave home without it) goes on my bedside table. If the room has a safe, I lock up several of my valuables when I'm not using them, but I still designate one drawer for the rest. This way I only need to pack Gigi's photo and go through that one drawer (and the safe) to avoid forgetting any valuables when I check out.

## Heading Off Forgetful Moments

Another common age-related memory annoyance involves forgetting something we had planned to do, or being unsure whether or not we have done something we were supposed to do. Who hasn't driven halfway to their destination and suddenly worried whether they'd fed the dog or turned off the coffee maker? No problem, you'll just call your wife and have her do it. Maybe she hasn't left the house yet. You search for your cell phone, rifling through your pockets and briefcase, finally pulling over and dumping it out completely on the seat beside you. Great, you forgot your phone.

Developing good memory habits can help you head off these kinds of forgetful moments and related memory panics. If you make a conscious effort to think about what you are doing while you're doing it, you are more likely to remember the action later. Some people even say out loud what they are doing while they do it, although if you try that method, you may want to check that no one is within earshot, or at least pretend to be talking into your phone or Bluetooth. If you have a tendency to leave your cell phone at home, create a memory place for it by always charging it overnight right next to your briefcase or purse.

To prevent the problem of forgetting plans and appointments, spend a few moments each morning reviewing your calendar for the day. I usually do this just after waking up by checking the calendar in my cell phone. I recommend that you always pick the same time and place for reviewing your upcoming day. After a week or so, it will become a memory habit that will help you avoid forgetting future plans. I also find it helpful to carry a to-do list with me at work. Then I check off small tasks, such as calls I had to make, after I've completed them.

## Pulling That Word Off the Tip of Your Tongue

One of the most frustrating memory challenges is when you know a word, name, or title, but it just won't come to mind. Despite your best efforts, you just can't pull out the word. A lot has been written about this tip-of-the-tongue phenomenon, but most people don't have a systematic approach to deal with it. Often we remember the word or name later, when we're not trying so hard to retrieve it.

While we are struggling with these word-finding delays, we tend to focus on associations to what we wish to recall, hoping these associations will help us find the word, such as "it's the movie with George Clooney and that new actress." Sometimes the memory neighborhoods in our brains get these associations to work, but not always, and pushing ourselves too much can cause anxiety, which only worsens the problem.

I've found the following strategies to be effective in minimizing tip-of-the-tongue memory challenges:

1. Jot down associations that relate to the word or phrase you are searching for.

2. If the word comes to you later—as it often does—write it down next to your associations. If it doesn't, you can keep exercising your brain while trying to come up with it on your own, or look up the word or phrase on the Internet or ask somebody.

3. Use *LOOK, SNAP, CONNECT* to link the word or phrase to your associations.

Here's an example of how it works. You see an ad for a Jeremy Irons film, and you mention to your friend how you've always thought he was a great actor, especially in that movie where he played those twin brothers. You know the one . . . it was really creepy. They were both gynecologists and they were addicted to drugs. Wasn't the word *twin* in the title? *Twin Peaks*? No, that wasn't it. Wait a minute, you'll think of it in a second . . .

On a notepad or in your phone, jot down Jeremy Irons—creepy twin gynecologist movie. When you get home, search online for Jeremy Irons movies and you'll find your sought-after title, *Dead Ringers*. Now visualize a snap of Jeremy Irons playing dead with a gold ring on each of his fingers. You'll probably never forget that title again. Even though the moment has passed when you really want to think of that movie title, and perhaps it's not likely to come again soon, using this method strengthens your brain so that you'll have fewer tip-of-the-tongue moments in the future.

## The Roman Room Method

Most of us have heard of memory savants who can recall amazing amounts of detailed information after just a quick glance. In 2010, Wang Feng won the World Memory Championships when he correctly memorized the order of 52 shuffled playing cards in less than 30 seconds. Like most memory masters, Mr. Feng likely used a trick that has been around for thousands of years: the Roman Room Method, named for the Roman orators who used the strategy to keep track of the ideas they wished to cover during their speeches. The technique is still used to overcome many memory challenges.

**TRY THIS!**

Use chunking (see p. 58) to memorize a phone number that you don't know by heart and need to look up.

Here's how it works. Begin by visualizing a familiar group of rooms, perhaps your apartment or house. In your mind, take a virtual stroll through the rooms. It's best if you take the same pathway through the rooms each time. Next, mentally place an image or snap that represents an idea, person, thing, or word that you want to remember in each room as you take another virtual stroll through your home.

For practice, let's say you are planning to give a toast at your daughter's wedding. You don't want to forget to mention anyone important, especially those new in-laws who took for granted that they could stay at your house the whole wedding weekend. You decide on everyone you are going to mention, perhaps jot their names down, and then begin your mental stroll. You start by mentally walking into the den and imagining that you see those in-laws there: The father's got his feet on your coffee table and he's smoking one of your best cigars, while the mother's busy disorganizing your meticulously alphabetized DVD collection. You move on to the kitchen and there's your future son-in-law at the open refrigerator, drinking milk straight from the carton. You enter the dining room and see your beautiful wife setting a lovely table. Finally you knock on your daughter's door and she opens it, looking like the most beautiful bride in the world.

Sure, you still have to write the toast, or perhaps wing it, but if you take your mind on a quick stroll through your house, you'll remember whom to mention and in the right order. You'll find that you can readily retrieve the *SNAP*s on future mental walks, and you'll probably remember that toast forever. The method works for almost anything—lists, errands, presentations, and lectures. You can add more rooms, more houses, estates, compounds, and before you know it, you can remember much more than you ever imagined.

You can take the Roman Room Method to Las Vegas or Atlantic City and start counting cards. Each card and suit will need a visual symbol that reminds you of the card and will be easy to remember with a little practice (for example, a *fork* can represent a *four* and a *tent* can be a *ten*). The dealer throws down the queen of hearts and you begin your stroll in your master bedroom, seeing a queen holding a valentine. You proceed to the hallway and bump into a diamond ring atop a large eight-ball (eight of diamonds). On the patio, you spot two garden spades (two of spades). Before you know it, you'll be beating the casino, or getting kicked out if the management figures out you're counting.

## Your Memory Has Already Improved

Even if you don't remember everything in this chapter, if you're trying some of these techniques, your memory ability has probably already improved. These methods are even more effective when combined with physical conditioning, a healthy brain diet, and relaxation techniques. Whether you use *LOOK, SNAP, CONNECT*, the Roman Room Method, chunking, or simply better observation skills, you'll find that memory training is an integral component of your Alzheimer's prevention program.

"MY GRANDMOTHER,
SHE STARTED WALKING FIVE
MILES A DAY WHEN SHE WAS SIXTY.
SHE'S NINETY-SEVEN TODAY
AND WE DON'T KNOW WHERE
THE HELL SHE IS."

—ELLEN DEGENERES

## CHAPTER 4

# Physical Exercise Protects the Brain

SOON AFTER TAKING ON A NEW JOB AS CEO of a technology company, Richard W. consulted with me about his memory concerns. He always felt he had an incredible, almost photographic memory for people's names, but now that he was 54, he was having trouble learning the names of his new staff. He'd read a lot about

Alzheimer's in the news and was worried that his memory changes might be the early symptoms of the disease.

We reviewed his medical and lifestyle background. Richard was in good health, his blood pressure and cholesterol levels were normal, and he was taking very few medicines. He had no family history of dementia, but his father had died of a heart attack at age 66. Although Richard felt some stress about his new high-level position, it wasn't affecting his sleep or his appetite. He ate a healthy diet and maintained an active social life. He did mention that since taking on the new job, he rarely had enough time for the daily tennis, jogging, or swimming that he used to do.

Besides the memory exercises I gave him, I recommended that Richard get back into his exercise routine. Regular cardiovascular conditioning would not only protect his heart, but it would be good for his brain, potentially improving his memory and lowering his future risk for Alzheimer's disease.

A month later, Richard returned to my office and said that he had gone back to running three miles every morning and playing tennis twice a week. He felt a lift in his mood and energy level, and his memory had definitely improved—he felt like his old photographic memory for names was coming back to him.

Physical activity gets us into shape, helps take off excess weight, and keeps us feeling young. I remember back in high school, the PE coach made us do hundreds of jumping jacks, sit-ups, and laps around the track. We reluctantly ran the tedious laps and moaned about it the whole time. The coach told us to stop complaining, because it was good for our hearts.

What we didn't know then—and many people still don't realize—is that those laps and jumping jacks were protecting not just our hearts but our brains, as well. The physical conditioning we were getting five days a week helped improve our mood and memory ability, increase our life expectancy, and reduce our risk for developing Alzheimer's disease in the future.

Swedish scientists have found an association between cardiovascular fitness and intelligence. They reported that the fitness habits of 18-year-olds predicted their educational achievements years later in life. A 2010 report from the Framingham Longitudinal Study confirmed many earlier studies indicating that moderate physical activity protects brain health. Daily brisk walks led to a 40 percent lower risk for developing Alzheimer's disease or any kind of dementia.

## Keep Walking to Stay Sharp

Gigi's Grandma Ollie lived in a third-floor walk-up apartment in the Upper West Side of New York City. Every day she went down those stairs several times to go to the post office or the cleaners and do a little grocery shopping, and, of course, she'd walk back up several times. She never forgot a birthday, an anniversary, or any holiday. And, boy you didn't want to forget to send her a card or call her on her birthday. If you did forget, you'd hear about it for a long time. She lived beyond 100 (although she only admitted to being 98).

GRANDMA OLLIE

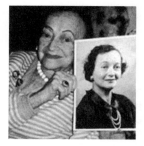

GRANDMA OLLIE: 103 years old, holding a photo of herself from her younger days.

Walking is one of the safest and most convenient ways to get an aerobic workout. How much walking or exercise each person needs depends on their baseline fitness level, age, and other health factors. However, becoming a weekend warrior who gets lots of exercise, but only on Saturday and Sunday, is not as effective as getting even short periods of cardio workouts throughout the week.

In a study of more than 18,000 older women, Harvard researchers found that a total of 90 minutes a week of brisk walking, or approximately 15 minutes a day, was all that was needed to delay cognitive decline and reduce possible risk for future Alzheimer's disease. University of Pittsburgh scientists found that the more that older people walk, the

69

better their cognitive abilities and the larger their brains, and larger brain size is associated with a lower risk for Alzheimer's disease.

Many studies have demonstrated that a lower risk for Alzheimer's disease is associated with almost any form of physical activity, whether it's gardening, housework, swimming, or tennis. When sedentary people start a fitness program, their brains grow larger in key memory regions such as the frontal lobe and hippocampus.

Q: **Does any kind of exercise help keep your brain healthy or do I have to do power walks, which I find boring?**

A: Most of the studies showing brain health benefits from physical exercise have involved walking as the primary intervention. However, any form of cardiovascular conditioning has similar effects on increasing brain blood flow and endorphin release. Newer studies also show that strength training can improve cognitive function and brain health as well. So if walking bores you, consider swimming, cycling, competitive sports, or any form of physical exercise you enjoy. The elliptical machine or any of the machines at the gym that provide a cardiovascular workout would have the same effect on boosting your heart and brain health.

Equally convincing evidence of the brain benefits of physical exercise comes from studies that have enrolled and monitored volunteers in exercise programs and compared them to sedentary control groups. Dr. Arthur Kramer and colleagues at the University of Illinois recruited volunteers aged 58 to 77 years and assigned them to either a walking group or a group that did stretching and toning. After six months the walkers had increased blood flow in brain circuits that control spatial ability and complex thinking, but the stretching and toning control group showed no such change. Although stretching and toning are important components of a comprehensive physical fitness program, Professor Kramer's findings demonstrate the added value of cardiovascular conditioning for maintaining brain health. Other research indicates that just 20 minutes of daily aerobic exercise can improve memory ability, and these improvements were still observed a year after completion of the initial physical training even when the daily exercise regimen is not maintained.

I not only feel energized and mentally sharp after a brisk walk, swim, or workout at the gym; I can almost beat Gigi at Scrabble (even *almost* is hard to do). Aerobic conditioning may be improving my memory and mental acuity in several ways. Exercise gets the heart pumping more blood, not just to the muscles but also to the brain. This added blood flow in the brain appears to reverse cellular deterioration associated with aging. It also stimulates the growth of new synapses, the connection sites between neurons, and makes brain cells more responsive to external stimuli. Studies of small animals have shown that exercise increases growth of brain blood vessels that deliver oxygen, as well as brain-derived neurotrophic factor (BDNF), a protein that stimulates brain cell growth and synaptic connections, leading to a more efficient, sensitive, and adaptive brain. BDNF is also associated with reduced risk for Alzheimer's disease.

## Pumping Iron Builds Brain Muscle

Most of us have seen body builders who lift huge barbells to enlarge their muscles and sculpt their bodies. They're usually trying to build larger biceps, washboard abs, and stronger hamstrings. Neuroscientists are now finding that this same kind of strength and resistance training also boosts brain fitness.

In one recent investigation, Brazilian researchers studied three groups of laboratory rats over eight weeks: a strength-training group that had tiny weights tied to their tails while they climbed little ladders; an aerobics group that ran on miniature treadmills; and a control group that essentially sat around. Both the strength-training and aerobic groups demonstrated improved learning and memory abilities. They also had higher levels of the protein BDNF. The sitting-around group's brains just "sat around" and showed no improvement.

Japanese researchers increased the resistance of the running wheels of laboratory animals similarly to the way we adjust the resistance on our treadmills or stationary bicycles. As a result of their increased resistance training (compared to a standard-issue running wheel exercise), the animals' DNA switched on to produce higher levels of BDNF. Thus, physical resistance exercise may not only build muscle strength but also turn on our genes to spark neuronal activity.

In studies of older women at the University of British Columbia, Dr. Teresa Liu-Ambrose found that weight lifters have better cognitive abilities than those who stick to only stretching and toning routines. Strength training seems to improve specific brain functions involving complex reasoning and attention skills that are controlled in the frontal lobe. Pumping iron builds brain muscle by increasing the heart's efficiency in supplying blood to the brain. The need to attend to form and technique while weight training may also provide a cognitive challenge not practiced when just stretching or running laps around the track.

## Does Exercise Cure Depression?

After just a few weeks of working out and playing tennis, our technology CEO, Richard W., noticed that his mood had lifted. Anyone who has run a 10-K or done any kind of rigorous training knows firsthand the immediate sense of endorphin-induced euphoria. We feel uplifted and clearheaded, and recent research suggests that it may have a lasting effect on relieving symptoms of depression.

Depression can distract us and impair our memory ability. It can also be one of the first symptoms of the onset of Alzheimer's disease in older adults. During our UCLA studies we have found that some symptoms of depression and even anxiety appear to correlate with the accumulation of amyloid plaques and tau tangles in the brain as Alzheimer's disease progresses.

Colleagues from Duke University recently compared the antidepressant effects of aerobic exercise training to the antidepressant sertraline (Zoloft), as well as a placebo pill. After four months, they found that exercise was just as good as or better than the Zoloft in treating depression. Those who exercised at a moderate level—about 40 minutes three to five days each week—experienced the greatest antidepressant effect.

Exercise not only releases endorphins, the body's own natural antidepressant, but it also releases the brain messenger serotonin, which elevates mood. Many of today's antidepressants like Zoloft or fluoxetine (Prozac) are SSRIs (selective serotonin reuptake inhibitors) that exert their effects on the brain's chemistry by increasing the amount of serotonin, a chemical that is decreased in depression. So the fitness component of your Alzheimer's prevention program may not only help your memory but also give you a boost in your mood.

## Getting Off the Couch

One night I set my alarm to go off early so I could get 20 minutes in on the treadmill before work. The next thing I knew, the alarm was blaring and I hit the snooze button for just a few more minutes of rest. Once I got out of bed, I figured a cup of coffee and the newspaper would be nice before my workout. The crossword puzzle looked sort of easy. I finished the puzzle and went to the closet to grab my sneakers, which I couldn't find in the mess of shoes. I started reorganizing my shoes, and then noticed the pile of wrinkled sweaters on the shelf above, so I began refolding them. OCD? Maybe, but I suddenly looked at my watch and realized that I would be late for work if I didn't skip the treadmill and get in the shower, asap. Maybe I'd work out tonight . . .

Now I almost always get my daily workout in. For most of us, the hardest part of an exercise program is getting started. But once we make it a habit and start seeing results, it becomes easier to stick with it. So, if we all know that exercise is good for our hearts and life expectancy, why doesn't everybody run ten miles a week? And with new discoveries showing how exercise protects the brain and potentially guards us from Alzheimer's disease, shouldn't there be a stampede to the running track?

One reason that everyone doesn't hop on the treadmill right now is that in general, most people don't put as much value on things that are down the road in the future. Our brains are hardwired for instant gratification. We want what's in front of us right now, especially if it looks, feels, or tastes good. The idea of having to work for something that we can get or achieve in the future—like a buffed-up body or a plumper frontal lobe—often seems theoretical and remote, even if it's only a week or two away.

Research from economist George Loewenstein at Carnegie Mellon University has shown that most people would sooner make a quick buck than wait to grow rich later. His team offered volunteers of all ages a choice between receiving $20 right away or waiting six months and receiving $110. Most of the research subjects opted for the quick cash. When neuroscientists peer into the brains of people making such choices, it's clear that the arousal state of the instant reward is much greater than that of waiting for a future payoff.

The good news is that physical exercise does provide instant gratification. The endorphin burst is immediate and makes us feel good. Taking a walk outside in the fresh air is usually invigorating and uplifting. Competitive sports such as basketball and tennis are exciting and fun and provide excellent aerobic workouts. The hurdle is getting ourselves to step up to the plate and take that first swing.

By integrating physical exercise seamlessly into your day, you get to feel that endorphin high without much effort. And after just a week or so, you may see other results, including a firmer body, increased energy, and possible weight loss.

## Aerobic Workouts That Go to Your Head

Aerobic conditioning is an essential component of any Alzheimer's prevention program. Whether you're climbing stairs or swimming laps, the goal is to get your heart pumping faster so it can deliver more oxygen and nutrients to your brain.

The key is to start at your baseline conditioning level and gradually build from there. As you increase your endurance, your heart and lungs become more efficient—you can work out longer with less effort—and your brain reaps the benefits of your having a more efficient heart.

I find it helpful to set small, achievable goals for myself, perhaps adding two blocks to my morning walk or slightly increasing the incline on my treadmill by one or two clicks. Achieving these minor milestones motivates me to push forward. As a workout becomes part of your daily routine, the efficiency of your heart, lungs, and circulatory system increases. Also, you'll lower your risk for high blood pressure, diabetes, and other age-related diseases that can damage brain neurons, and the calories you burn will help control your weight.

Your workout sessions don't have to last for hours: Even small bursts of exertion are health promoting. Systematic studies have found that multiple periods of brief exercise—three 10-minute sessions spread throughout the day—can be as effective in controlling weight and lowering risk for heart disease as a single half-hour session.

Start with a warmup phase to raise your body temperature and loosen your joints. This will increase your pulse and prepare your heart for a more vigorous workout. After an aerobics session, take a few moments to cool down and gradually bring your body back to its resting state. Stretch your muscles to keep them limber, minimize soreness, and increase your flexibility.

The following are examples of some aerobic workouts. Which type of conditioning you choose will depend on convenience and what fits best with your current lifestyle. Since the brain craves variety, try switching up your exercise routines now and then.

---

**AEROBIC WORKOUTS**

TAKE A WALK. Whether you're walking on the treadmill or the sidewalk or even at the mall, it's good for you. It's more difficult on the sand at the beach, but if I'm forced to walk on the beach of a beautiful tropical island, I guess I can make myself do it.

Many baby boomers have experienced their fair share of aches and pains, bad knees, and ruptured discs, making it difficult to jog or run for fitness. Today we know that walking at a brisk pace is just as good for your brain and body as running and poses minimal risk for injury.

I live in the hills, and on the weekends I like to park my car at the bottom of my hill and do my errands on foot. That way I get my afternoon walk in and take care of my tasks at the same time. Some people like to wear a pedometer so they can keep track of just how much they've walked and how many calories they've burned. I've tried this, but I tend to stare at the pedometer and run the risk of bumping into trees and people.

Whenever there's enough time, my walks become a family outing that includes the dog, and I get a chance to hear my teenagers moan about the hills and ask incessantly when we are going to turn around and go home. Scaling hills can be a great way to build stamina and increase your heart rate.

CYCLING. An estimated one out of every three people age 65 or older suffers from knee or ankle pain, and those sore joints have led many of them to try cycling. The smooth, circular movement of cycling not only provides an aerobic challenge, but it can even strengthen knee joints. Outdoor cycling is a great way to get some fresh air, but it should always be done while wearing a helmet. Protecting our heads from injury is crucial for lowering our risk for Alzheimer's disease. If weather or local terrain prevents outdoor biking, a stationary bike or elliptical machine offers a good alternative, and you can watch the news or read a book while working out. Another plus of the stationary bike is you don't have to mess up your hair with a helmet.

SWIMMING. I love swimming because it not only offers a great cardiovascular workout, but it engages almost every major muscle group in the body. Because it is a non-weight-bearing exercise, it is ideal for people who have suffered joint injuries from higher-impact cardiovascular workouts. You can start with just a few laps and build up your stamina over time. If you have an injury, you can easily vary the strokes and kicks to avoid overworking a particular muscle group or joint.

RACQUET SPORTS. Competitive sports like tennis and racquet-ball are great ways to motivate us to get physical. With racquet sports, you're not just achieving an aerobic workout, but the mental challenge strengthens three major brain areas that control hand-eye coordination, movement, and balance. Even table tennis offers these benefits. Chess provides a mental challenge as well, but you usually don't get much of a cardiovascular burn, unless, of course, you pace a lot between turns.

GETTING FIT AND TIDY AT THE SAME TIME. I occasionally do a little work around the house (Gigi would say *very* occasionally). Epidemiological studies have found a link between a lower risk for Alzheimer's disease and almost anything that picks up your breathing rate and the pace of your heart. Raking leaves in the yard, sweeping the floors, and cleaning out the attic involve lifting, bending, and other movements that can give you a pretty good workout. Chores burn calories, too: In just 10 minutes you can burn off 50 calories by hedging the bushes or about 75 calories by mowing the lawn. (Using a riding mower doesn't count.)

CUT A RUG. Dancing combines aerobic physical activity with emotional and sensory stimulation, social interaction, and motor coordination—what scientists would call an enriched environmental condition. Brain scans of experienced dancers show strengthened neural circuits in regions involved in motor control, as well as greater neuroplasticity in their brains compared with the brains of novice dancers. Ruhr-University scientists in Germany found that people age 65 and older who had an average of nearly 17 years of amateur dancing under their belts had significantly better cognitive, motor, and perceptual abilities than a nondancing control group.

WALK THE DOG. Getting a person off the couch and on to the treadmill is one thing—keeping him off the couch is quite another. Investigators at the University of Missouri College of Veterinary Medicine found that the answer can be as simple as getting a dog. Having a dog motivates people to start walking and stick with it. After all, Rover needs his exercise, even if you don't feel like getting any. The adherence rate to a regular walking program over a period of 50 weeks was 72 percent for dog walkers, who also experienced an average weight loss of more than 14 pounds. I have a dog. He loves to walk, and he's already lost about 8 pounds.

SHOP TO EXERCISE YOUR BRAIN. Many people love to shop (you know who you are). Going shopping combines physical exercise like walking between stores and perhaps trying on hundreds of pairs of shoes, with brain activities ranging from searching through sale items to choosing colors and figuring out what 30 percent off equals. Although shopping may do damage to your credit cards, it can be good for your brain, since it provides exercise and activates brain centers that control memory, planning, and visual and spatial skills. And don't forget the social interaction you get when surrounded by sales people oohing and aahing at your fabulous choices.

## Strength and Resistance Training

For years I've known about the heart and brain benefits of aerobic conditioning. With the latest scientific evidence now also pointing to the cognitive benefits of weight-lifting and resistance training, I joined a gym and have begun building up my muscles. I'm certainly no Mr. America, but I feel stronger, and I know I'm protecting my brain. I now alternate my aerobic workouts with weight and resistance training. Taking a breather from the treadmill every other day has delighted my middle-aged knees.

Resistance and strength training not only protects brain health and builds muscle mass, but it helps make bones denser and lowers our risk for osteoporosis, which can make bones more brittle with age, so that a fall or trauma is more likely to cause a fracture. Strength training also helps stabilize blood sugar levels, which can protect us from diabetes. Most people think of weight lifting as a sport reserved for young, buffed, muscle-bound athletes, but research shows that older people, even those in their eighties, benefit from pumping iron.

At every age, it's important to train opposing muscle groups, biceps and triceps, for instance, to reduce the risk of injuries. When beginning weight training, start out with light weight, then as your strength increases, build up both your repetitions and the amount of weight you lift. That way, you'll avoid injury and achieve reasonable goals. As much as I'd like to be able to bench press 200 pounds today, it doesn't happen overnight. For me, it probably won't happen in my lifetime, but I can dream.

Strength training tears down muscle fiber, but cross training—working different muscle groups on alternate days—allows these muscle groups to rest between training sessions so they can repair and rebuild. One day you might work out your upper body muscles (arms, shoulders, back, and chest), while the following day you could focus on your lower body (thighs, calves, and hamstrings). You could also do weight training one day and switch to aerobic conditioning the next. Consider the following strength-training exercises for building up your body and your brain.

WORKING WITH WEIGHTS. Training with free weights can work out muscles from many angles in order to isolate and strengthen specific muscle groups. Working out with a trainer or someone with experience can help you learn correct form so your workout is injury-free and you develop control, balance, and coordination. If you work out in a gym, you can achieve similar benefits with weight-lifting equipment. The machines guide the weight-lifting motions and reinforce correct posture. Tips from a trainer may also increase the effectiveness of a machine workout and reduce your risk for injury.

RESISTANCE AND ISOMETRIC EXERCISES. Exercise bands, available at drugstores or sporting goods stores, come in varying degrees of resistance and can be used to work out upper- and lower-body muscle groups. If you don't have an assortment of bands, you can wrap or double your available band to make it tighter and increase its resistance as you get stronger. Since elastic bands are light in weight, they are easy to pack and great for keeping up your exercise program when you travel. Stand on the center of your band and you can work your biceps by doing curls, or your shoulders by lifting your arms straight out laterally. If you hold the band behind your back and lift the opposite end above your head with the other hand, you can work your triceps (see figures).

Without a band, you can do isometric exercises, which involve muscular contractions with resistance and no movement. Here is an example of a simple

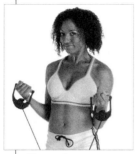

Biceps curls

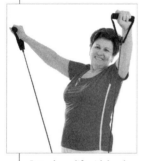

Lateral arm lift with band

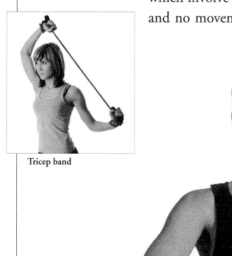

Tricep band

Isometric

isometric exercise that will strengthen your upper body (biceps, triceps, and chest): Sit up straight and push your hands together in front of your chest. Breathe slowly and deeply and hold for five seconds, then rest between reps.

## Balance and Stability

Balance and stability become increasingly important for maintaining body and brain health as we age. Older research volunteers who incorporate balance training in their exercise programs show significant improvements in memory and other cognitive abilities. Good balance and stability help prevent injuries from falls. Head trauma that causes loss of consciousness for an hour or more doubles the risk for developing Alzheimer's disease.

Exercises that improve balance stimulate brain neural circuits to send messages from the brain to the body, making it better able to right itself if it becomes unsteady. These neural networks inform us how to react and how much tension is needed in each muscle group in order to remain upright. The brain health benefits from balance and stability exercises could result, in part, from this focused form of cognitive training.

Balance and stability training doesn't have to involve elaborate equipment. Standing on one leg and looking in the mirror is a simple and effective training exercise. Start out for a count of 5 to 10. Once you are able to remain balanced for 30 seconds on each leg, try doing it with your eyes closed. It may be a lot harder, but with practice you can work toward that goal. Here are some other ways to improve your balance and stability.

Standing on one leg

81

DANCING. Dancing not only offers aerobic conditioning benefits, but it also helps people keep balanced. Investigators at Aristotle University of Thessaloniki, in Greece, assessed the effect of a ten-week traditional Greek dance program on objective measures of balance in healthy older adults. They found that the dance group showed significant improvements in balance when standing and moving compared with a control group. Other studies have found that older adults who are regular social dancers have better balance and stability when standing or walking compared with nondancers. So whether you like to cha-cha, rumba, or mambo, it can be a way to have fun while improving your balance and stability.

TAI CHI. This popular Eastern practice uses slow and smooth movements that offer several brain health benefits. The meditative component reduces stress, while the slow, deliberate movements improve cardiovascular conditioning, balance, and stability. The process of learning the exercises and maintaining proper form likely activates specialized neural circuits that provide a brain exercise.

PILATES. This exercise system was developed by Joseph Pilates as a way for people to increase strength, flexibility, and coordination. It incorporates controlled movements that strengthen the body's core muscles, including the stomach, lower back, buttocks, and inner thighs. These muscle groups provide the body's structural support, which maintains our balance and stability. A recent study found that middle-aged people who attended a 12-week Pilates class for an hour twice weekly showed significant improvement in objective measures of balance and posture compared with a control group. Although a full Pilates program requires the assistance of an instructor and special Pilates equipment, simpler exercises based on the same principles can be done on your own.

BALANCE BALLS. Years ago when our kids were little, I walked into my bedroom and saw a giant orange ball on the floor at the far corner of the bed. It looked like a small orange planet. I noticed my wife's feet sticking out from behind the bed, balancing on the ball, pulling it in toward her and then pushing it away.

"What are you doing with that? Is it one of the kids' toys?" She shushed me and said she was working on her glutes.

Today, I know lots of ways to use the balance ball for stretching, core strengthening, and balance and stability training. By introducing an element of instability into any exercise, which the balance ball does, it challenges us to strengthen muscle groups in addition to the ones the exercise was intended to work. Researchers at Bond University, in Australia, found that balance ball training led to significant improvements in lower back muscle endurance and flexibility, leg strength, and balance.

## Keeping Fitness Fun and Safe

Wear and tear over the years makes our bodies more vulnerable to injuries, so we need to be more cautious and creative in achieving fitness goals and keeping our exercises safe than when we were young. Specific exercises to strengthen certain vulnerable body areas can make a big difference. Below are a few exercises and stretches that I've found helpful in strengthening my core muscles (which protect my back) and improving my balance and flexibility. They don't require any equipment, so you can do them anywhere.

ABDOMINAL CRUNCH. Lie on your back with your knees bent and feet flat on the floor. As you exhale, tighten your abdomen by pulling your belly button in and pushing it toward your chin. Inhale deeply. Place your hands behind your head and as you exhale and pull your belly button in and tighten your abdominal muscles—that's the "crunch"

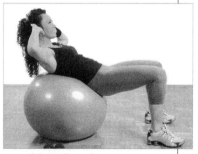

Abdominal crunch on balance ball

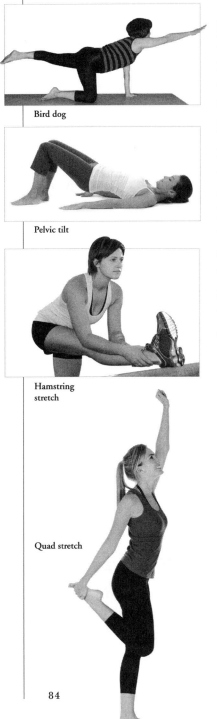

Bird dog

Pelvic tilt

Hamstring
stretch

Quad stretch

part—pull your torso toward the ceiling. Do not pull your neck and head up with your hands, but lift them up with the muscles of your upper body. To make it harder, try the crunches while your back is supported by a balance ball (see photo, p. 83).

BIRD DOG. Get on your hands and knees, with your hands directly below your shoulders and your knees bent at 90 degrees. Keep your back flat, your stomach pulled up, and your head level and even with your spine. Point your right arm straight forward and your left leg straight back. Hold for 5 seconds, gradually building up to 30 seconds. Then switch sides. Repeat 5 times.

Side stretch

SIDE STRETCH. Stand with your feet shoulder width apart. Raise your right arm over your head and, keeping your shoulders, hips, and knees aligned, lean to the left until you feel your right-side muscles stretching. Hold for 5 seconds and then do the opposite side. Repeat for a total of 10 stretches.

PELVIC TILT. Lie on your back with your knees bent and feet flat on the floor. Lift your pelvis off the floor while tightening your buttocks for a count of five, then roll down. Repeat 10 times.

HAMSTRING STRETCH. Stand in front of a chair, table, or wall and rest your right heel on the surface. Keeping both legs straight, lean forward until you feel a stretch in your hamstring. Hold for 10 seconds. Repeat on the other side.

QUAD STRETCH. Standing with your knees parallel, lift your right foot toward your buttocks. Grab your foot with your right hand and hold for 10 seconds. Now do the other side. If you need to, hold on to a chair or table and steady yourself with your opposite hand.

These are only a few examples of the many stretches and exercises you can do to stay fit and prevent injury. As much as possible, look for opportunities throughout your day when you can add an extra pop of cardiovascular work, such as taking the stairs instead of the elevator or walking briskly to a nearby errand instead of driving the car. You can also try jumping jacks in the restroom, jogging to get your mail, or doing the twist while washing the dishes. Making their regular workout a social event motivates a lot of people to stick with their fitness programs. It doesn't have to be a competitive sport like tennis or basketball—it can be an invigorating power walk with a friend, around the neighborhood or on tandem treadmills at the fitness center. Keeping the body healthy through exercise is an essential part of any Alzheimer's prevention program.

"I STAY AWAY FROM
NATURAL FOODS.
AT MY AGE
I NEED ALL THE
PRESERVATIVES I CAN GET."
—George Burns

## CHAPTER 5

# Healthy
# Brain
# Nutrition

CAROLYN B. HAD STRUGGLED WITH HER WEIGHT since she was in her teens, and now that she had teenagers of her own, she still struggled with it. If she could just drop 15 pounds, she'd be ecstatic. Carolyn had tried every fad diet out there, but even when she did lose a few pounds, she just put them right back on again.

Her marketing job was busy and stressful, so she didn't always have time to grab the healthiest lunches. And racing home to get dinner on the table for her husband and kids didn't lend itself to preparing low-calorie, healthy meals every night. But she was trying. She resisted the chips that came with her sandwich at lunch, and she ate salads whenever she could. She had thrown out her bathroom scale because weighing herself every morning just made her obsess more about food. Even though she was heavier than she wanted to be, she actually felt pretty good.

When Carolyn went for her yearly medical check-up, she got quite a surprise—she'd put on ten pounds since her last visit. Ten pounds! That was crazy! But then she thought about the vending machine candy bars that she sneaked at work when she got stressed out, and the late-night cracker binges she had while watching TV after her husband fell asleep. Okay, everybody has a slip once in a while . . . but ten pounds? And now her doctor mentioned his concern about possible diabetes. That really scared her.

Her doctor explained that people with diabetes have abnormally high levels of sugar or glucose in their blood. They often need medicine to regulate it, but exercise and diet could help control it, too. Without treatment, diabetes could be dangerous and increase her risk for Alzheimer's and other age-related diseases.

Carolyn left in a daze. Diabetes? Alzheimer's disease? It made her head spin, and she felt like stopping at the next corner and eating five hotdogs. But she didn't. Never mind looking better, her doctor was talking about serious illnesses here. If she had ever been motivated to do something about her eating habits, it was now.

The key to good nutrition is not just going on a diet, it is changing the way we think about food. Like many people, Carolyn spent a lot of time and energy focusing on how her body weight made her look, and this preoccupation was tied up with her self-esteem. Her doctor finally got through to her that what she ate didn't just affect her appearance, but it also had an impact on her risk for various diseases. Carolyn started to rethink her old ways of planning, preparing, and eating meals. She was no longer just trying to lose weight. She had a new goal now—to eat the kinds of foods that would protect her body and her brain, and she was determined to make sure her family ate those foods, too.

Eating a healthy diet means getting the right vitamins and nutrients to nourish the organs and cells of the body. Scientific evidence points to some foods that promote brain health and others that are best to avoid. A recent Columbia University study of more than 2,000 people age 65 and older found a lower risk for Alzheimer's disease in the volunteers who ate the greater amount of nuts, fish, tomatoes, poultry, vegetables, and fruits, and the lesser amount of high-fat dairy products, red meat, and butter. This and many other studies show that nutritious meals can help prevent many common health problems that influence brain function and risk for Alzheimer's disease.

## Metabolic Syndrome and the Epidemic of Obesity

During the past two decades, the prevalence of obesity in the U.S. has risen dramatically. Today, nearly 73 million Americans are obese, and according to the Centers for Disease Control and Prevention, obesity is a particular problem for people age 50 and older. Being obese or overweight increases an individual's risk for heart disease, stroke, and diabetes. It also impairs brain health and increases the risk for developing Alzheimer's disease.

One out of every five obese individuals suffers from a symptom cluster known as the metabolic syndrome, characterized by extra weight around the middle of the body (central obesity); elevated blood sugar, triglycerides, and blood pressure; and low HDL "good" cholesterol levels. Compared to people with normal metabolic values, people with metabolic syndrome have a higher risk for developing heart disease and memory loss. In a four-year study of more than 7,000 French volunteers age 65 and older, high overall cholesterol levels or low levels of the healthy HDL cholesterol, hypertension, and high blood sugar levels were associated with greater cognitive impairment.

We can estimate ideal body weight by using our height and weight to calculate our body mass index, or BMI. Obesity is often defined as a BMI of 30 or more, whereas being overweight or preobese is usually a

BMI that ranges between 25 and 30. Healthy weight is a BMI under 25.

The following formula will help you calculate your BMI. If you would like to use your computer to make the calculation for you, visit www.cdc.gov and click on BMI Calculator.

### FORMULA FOR CALCULATING BMI

$$\text{BMI} = \frac{(\text{weight in pounds}) \times 703}{(\text{height in inches})^2}$$

In a study of more than 2,000 healthy individuals aged 32 to 62, scientists at Toulouse University, in France, found that a higher BMI at the beginning of the study was associated with greater cognitive decline five years later. People with high BMIs had trouble learning a list of words and in substituting numbers for symbols, a standard measure of how rapidly the brain can process information.

However, because BMI doesn't tell us where the fat is located, it doesn't give us the whole story. Some people can have a high BMI and still be at a healthy weight because they have more lean body mass than the average person. Also, there are middle-aged and older people with a normal BMI but very high amounts of body fat and low amounts of muscle mass. They may have central obesity and are at greater risk for metabolic syndrome.

The type of fat that expands our waistlines is no longer considered inert tissue for storing energy; it is quite active in regulating normal and abnormal body function. The cells, hormones, and other molecules produced and stored in the body's fat tissue around the middle, particularly in obese individuals, promotes insulin resistance—our cells become less responsive to insulin, a hormone that regulates the level of sugar in the body. Insulin resistance can lead to diabetes and increase the risk for cardiovascular disease. Researchers from Boston University School of Medicine found that in people at an average age of 60, the greater the degree of central obesity—regardless of overall body weight—the smaller the individual's brain size, and we know that smaller brain size heightens the risk for dementia.

Carolyn B. was concerned about gaining 10 pounds, and her worries were not unfounded. The sooner she shed her excess weight, the better, since the longer we carry around extra pounds, the harder it is to lose them. Neuroscientists have found evidence that as BMI rises, the ability to control appetite may decline, and neurons in the frontal lobe start functioning abnormally as BMI increases. It's no surprise that this frontal lobe is the brain region that modulates complex reasoning and impulse control.

## Manage Cravings: Use Your Imagination

I remember coming home from school sometimes when I was a kid to find my mother icing a chocolate cake she'd baked for dessert. That meant that no, I couldn't have a piece of that delicious-looking cake for my after-school snack; I'd have to wait centuries until after dinner, when she would finally allow us to have a slice. No amount of bargaining, or my reasonable arguments about why a slice right now would only show off how great the cake looked inside when she served it later, would change her mind. She told me to put the idea of eating the cake right out of my head. That's where my mother was wrong (sorry, Mom).

Our brains are constantly sending us signals about whether or not we're hungry, as well as what we're hungry for. When we crave unhealthy foods or even too much of a healthy food, we need to find ways to manage those brain signals. And sometimes the strategies for controlling cravings are counterintuitive.

A 2010 study published in *Science* magazine suggests that if we're craving a piece of chocolate cake, we should not try to distract ourselves from that urge, but instead focus our attention on eating a slice of chocolate cake. Scientists at Carnegie Mellon University assigned study subjects to three groups: One was instructed to imagine inserting coins into a laundry machine; a second was told to imagine inserting the coins and also eating three M&Ms; and a third was directed to imagine inserting the coins and eating 30 M&Ms. After these mental tasks were completed several times, the subjects were given a large number of M&Ms and told they could eat as many as they liked. The subjects who had imagined eating 30 M&Ms each time ate significantly fewer real M&Ms than the other groups. Apparently, by thinking about eating so many M&Ms already, they had had their fill. For this type of visualization to work, you have to be specific. If I daydream about M&Ms, I may eat fewer M&Ms but I'll still crave my chocolate cake. I also have to imagine actually eating the food. It won't work if I just imagine seeing the cake sitting on the counter.

**TRY THIS!**

Do you remember what you ate for dinner last night? Was it good for your brain? How about the night before that?

This mental exercise takes advantage of a brain process known as *habituation*. If we spend a lot of time thinking about eating M&Ms (or any craved food), the neural circuits involved in craving and eating M&Ms adapt and become bored by the *mere idea* of eating them, or perhaps the brain somehow comes to think that we have actually eaten what we're picturing. Essentially, the thrill is gone when it comes to the craved food.

Focusing attention on our meals while eating them can also help trim our waistlines. Researchers at the University of Bristol, in the UK, found that people who ate lunch while working or focusing on other activities felt less full afterward compared to those who ate the same meal but were not distracted while eating. Some of the distracted eaters also had trouble remembering what they had eaten. The bottom line is that concentrating on what we eat can help us control our cravings and feel more satisfied.

Researchers have now pinpointed a network of brain regions associated with satiation, which is that full feeling. They measured brain function in people who had distended stomachs from a small balloon that made them feel full. Functional MRI scans showed high activity in the amygdala, a brain region that controls many emotional reactions. They also found activity in the insula, an area that modulates physical sensations in the body. Volunteers with higher BMIs showed less activity in these brain regions while their stomachs were distended, which might explain why overweight and obese individuals have a harder time controlling food intake. Their brains are less responsive to neural signals from the stomach telling them it's time to stop eating.

## Calories Count

The professor in my pre-med physics class taught us that calories are simply units of energy and that losing weight followed a very easy formula: An individual merely needed to consume fewer calories than the number they burned off each day. Nutrition research since my Physics 101 class has confirmed this lesson—many comparisons of low-fat versus high-fat/high-protein diets don't seem to differ in their long-term weight-loss success rates. Mark Haub, a professor of human nutrition at Kansas State University, was dubbed the Twinkie Guy after he lost 27 pounds in less than three months on a diet consisting mostly of Twinkies.

To lose that much weight, he probably didn't eat very many Twinkies, and he must have felt pretty hungry most of the time. It's much easier to stay on a diet and control calories when we balance healthy and more satisfying carbohydrates and proteins. Some studies have found that very low carbohydrate diets are more effective than low-fat diets for short-term weight loss.

Avoiding excess calories, regardless of the actual food, is an important component of an Alzheimer's prevention program to elude the negative brain effects of weight-related illnesses such as diabetes and hypertension. And although bingeing on a couple of Twinkies once in a while can be fun, the fun doesn't last long and those empty calories don't provide your brain with any of the nutrients it needs to combat Alzheimer's disease. A diet that only forces you to avoid or forsake your favorite foods will make you feel deprived and less likely to stick with your program. Eating foods that meet your daily nutritional needs is critical for a healthy brain diet.

## Food Fight: Beating Inflammation

Inflammation is one of the first responses of the immune system, which is our body's defense mechanism that protects us from infections, foreign bodies, or other physical threats. When our immune system is out of whack, we are more susceptible to bacterial or viral infections. Being overweight throws off our immune system, but physical exercise and a healthy diet can help us lose excess weight and repair our immune system's functional integrity.

As scientists continue to figure out how the body ages, they are discovering that chronic inflammation is a driving force of many age-related illnesses—not only cancer and heart disease, but also Alzheimer's disease. When our body's immune system is working correctly, it helps the body heal from injuries, but too much of a good thing can cause problems over time.

Lack of sleep, stress, toxins such as smoke, and a sedentary lifestyle all contribute to chronic inflammation, and tiny proteins in the fat cells around the stomach (known as proinflammatory cytokines) trigger excess inflammation throughout the body. The good news is that nutritional scientists are discovering many foods that can help our bodies control inflammation and protect brain health. Some studies have indicated that a low-calorie diet can alter the expression of inflammatory genes in fat tissue. In other words, the number of calories we eat each day can have a direct effect on the DNA in fat cells. Ingesting fewer calories turns on anti-inflammatory genes to help control chronic inflammation.

Many of the foods in the Alzheimer's prevention diet, including fruits, vegetables, fish, whole grains, and legumes, fight inflammation. Spices and aromatic herbs also have anti-inflammatory effects and may boost immune function. In addition, a group of compounds known as flavonoids, present in colorful fruits and vegetables, have been found to protect the body from chronic inflammation.

# The Food–Mood Connection

Recently I was rushing between meetings and didn't have time for lunch. By 2:00 P.M. I was famished. I ran across the street to a market where they have ready-made hot foods and sandwiches. The first thing I saw was tempting—delicious-looking barbeque ribs, which I knew were going to be greasy and full of fat, but man, they smelled great. At the next counter, I saw Panini sandwiches with mozzarella cheese, sun-dried tomatoes, and basil. They didn't look as succulent as the ribs, but I grabbed the sandwich and ate it on the way to my next meeting. My hunger was satisfied, my mood was lifted, and I felt good about having made the right choice.

Food affects our mood in a variety of ways, but not all of the scientific theories about the food-mood connection have panned out. For example, we've been told that tryptophan in turkey will make us feel groggy, but the amount of turkey one would need to ingest in order to have a mental effect (about half of a 12-pound bird) wouldn't leave much for the rest of the family at Thanksgiving.

One consistent finding is that omega-3 fatty acids from foods like fish will stabilize mood and diminish depression. Multiple studies have shown that omega-3s have an antidepressant effect not only for people with mild depression but also for those with moderately severe depression. In fact, the American Psychiatric Association recommends that patients with major depression make sure they get enough omega-3 fat in their diet.

Scientists have noted an inverse correlation between the amount of fish consumed and the rates of depression in various countries around the world. In many Asian countries, where fish consumption is high, people are less likely to get depressed compared with the U.S. and Canada, where people eat less fish.

Someone who suffers from clinical depression should try to eat at least two 6-ounce servings of fish every week. It's also a good idea to avoid foods rich in omega-6 fatty acids, like corn and vegetable oils or processed foods, which can counteract the benefits of healthy brain omega-3s. Several fish are good sources of omega-3 fats, including wild (not farmed) salmon, trout, and tuna. Tilapia is not a good omega-3 source, and swordfish is best avoided because of its high mercury content. For more information on fish and omega-3, visit http://www.omega3oils.info/omega3sources/fishoil.php.

## Extra, Extra: Get Your Antioxidants

Eating antioxidant foods may protect our brains from oxidative free radicals that cause wear and tear on the DNA in our cells. Colorful berries, such as strawberries, blackberries, and blueberries contain polyphenols that fight oxidants. Antioxidant foods containing polyphenols include other fruits: grapes, pears, plums, and cherries; as well as vegetables: broccoli, cabbage, celery, onions, and parsley.

The Rotterdam Study, in the Netherlands, recently reported that higher dietary intake of the antioxidant vitamin E was associated with a lower risk for developing Alzheimer's disease. In another large-scale European study, of more than 8,000 volunteers age 65 and older, daily consumption of fruits and vegetables was associated with a decreased risk of all causes of dementia.

Low levels of antioxidants in the blood are associated with memory impairment, and laboratory animals fed antioxidant-rich berry extracts show better short-term memory (measured by how well they find their way through mazes). Other studies indicate that people who eat antioxidant fruits and vegetables have a lower risk for developing Alzheimer's disease.

Nutritional scientists use a standard measure that determines a food's ability to fight oxidation. This *Oxygen Radical Absorbency Capacity* (ORAC) score provides a general indication of how effective a particular food is at protecting brain cells from the damaging bombardment of free radicals. Most people eat only about 1,000 ORAC units a day, yet some experts recommend a daily dose closer to 3,500 units for optimal brain protection.

The table on page 97, based on laboratory measurements from the

U.S. Department of Agriculture, lists examples of some fruits and vegetables ranked according to their antioxidant potency.

I recommend eating a wide range of these foods, since each fruit and vegetable has its own unique nutrient profile. You can get an antioxidant boost by eating fruits and vegetables in a salad or snack, taking an antioxidant supplement, or drinking fruit and vegetable juices. Investigators from Vanderbilt School of Medicine, in Nashville, Tennessee, found that drinking fruit or vegetable juice at least three times a week compared with less than once a week lowered the risk for developing Alzheimer's disease.

Recent work from our UCLA research group showed that drinking pomegranate juice may provide an extra boost of brain power. We studied people aged 50 to 75 (average age 64) who had mild memory complaints associated with aging. Half the group drank an 8-ounce glass of pomegranate juice each day, while the other half drank 8 ounces of placebo drink that had the color and taste of pomegranate juice, but without the potent antioxidant polyphenol extracts contained in actual pomegranate juice. After a month, the volunteers who drank the pomegranate juice had significantly better memory scores. We also found that the pomegranate group showed a different pattern of brain activity while playing a videogame that required

## SOME POTENT ANTIOXIDANT FOODS

| FRUITS | ANTIOXIDANT POTENCY ORAC Units per 3½ Ounces |
|---|---|
| cranberries | 9,100 |
| prunes (dried plums) | 8,100 |
| plums | 7,600 |
| blackberries | 5,900 |
| raspberries | 5,100 |
| blueberries | 4,700 |
| pomegranates | 4,500 |
| strawberries | 4,300 |
| apples, Granny Smith | 3,900 |
| raisins | 3,400 |
| apricots, dried | 3,200 |
| apples, Gala | 2,800 |
| peaches | 1,900 |
| avocados, hass | 1,900 |
| oranges | 1,800 |
| red grapes | 1,800 |
| pears, red anjou | 1,700 |
| grapefruit | 1,600 |

| VEGETABLES | ANTIOXIDANT POTENCY ORAC Units per 3½ Ounces |
|---|---|
| garlic, raw | 5,700 |
| red cabbage, raw | 2,500 |
| sweet potato, baked with skin | 2,100 |
| broccoli, steamed | 2,100 |
| beets, raw | 1,800 |
| radishes | 1,700 |
| spinach, raw | 1,500 |
| red onions, raw | 1,500 |
| yellow onions, sautéed | 1,200 |
| romaine lettuce | 1,000 |

memory for places—their brain regions controlling visual and memory functions showed greater levels of activity.

Studies of small animals with the human Alzheimer's gene have demonstrated similar brain health benefits from pomegranate juice. Experimental Alzheimer's mice that drank pomegranate juice for six months had significantly better memory ability when finding their way through their mazes compared to those drinking placebo. The juice-drinking mice also had fewer amyloid plaques in their brains.

Most of us don't consume enough fruits and vegetables, and upping our servings is good not only for the brain but for the rest of the body, too. If you're concerned about the extra calories from raisins or prunes, green tea is another good source of antioxidants, and its phytochemicals have antiamyloid and anti-inflammatory properties as well. Choosing the right antioxidant vegetables will satiate those hunger pangs and help with weight control: Eight ounces of your favorite green leafy vegetable can fill you up more than your favorite processed cookie. Tomatoes contain a strong antioxidant known as lycopene, so V-8 and tomato juice are also good antioxidant options. And fresh is not the only way—frozen berries maintain their antioxidant power and make great healthy brain snacks.

## Good Fats, Bad Fats

When I was in grade school, a popular put-down was calling someone a fat-head. Little did we know that fat-head was actually a good thing, since our brains consist primarily of fat and having a bigger (fatter) brain could mean having a smarter brain.

Fat is essential to brain structure and function, but when it comes to healthy brain nutrition, the type of fat we ingest is just as important as the amount. Of course, eating too much of any kind of fat can lead to weight issues and obesity, but we need to learn to balance the good and bad fats.

Most of us have no problem getting enough of the bad fats—the omega-6 fats from bacon, burgers, steaks, margarine, mayonnaise, and most processed and fried foods, as well as corn and vegetable oils. These polyunsaturated omega-6 fats promote inflammation and contribute to brain cell damage if we overindulge in them over the years. A diet rich in omega-6 fats has been shown to impair memory in laboratory animals, and their brain neurons have fewer branches to connect with each other.

To protect our brains, we need to minimize our intake of omega-6 fats—say good-bye to the bacon, lamb chops, and butter cookies—and instead choose the grilled wild salmon as your entrée and perhaps grab a handful of walnuts as a snack. These substitutions are rich in omega-3 fatty acids that protect the heart and brain. Numerous studies have shown that people who consume large amounts of these anti-inflammatory omega-3 fatty acids have a lower risk of developing Alzheimer's disease. The most abundant omega-3 fatty acid in the brain, docosahexaenoic acid, or DHA, protects brain neurons against the damage associated with amyloid plaques and tau tangles. Studies comparing rates of dementia in Nigerians who eat a diet low in animal fat compared with African Americans whose diets have much more omega-6 fat show that the Nigerians have lower rates of Alzheimer's disease.

Substituting foods high in omega-3 fats or healthy monounsaturated fats (for example, olive or canola oil), for those high in omega-6 fats can also make us feel more satisfied and thus eat less, which helps control weight. One study of restaurant goers found that those given olive oil for their bread instead of butter ended up eating 23 percent less bread compared to those given butter.

Q: I heard that cooking with aluminum pots and pans can give you Alzheimer's disease. Is that true?

A: Autopsy studies have detected small deposits of aluminum in damaged areas of the brains of Alzheimer's patients, and some people have expressed concern that aluminum exposure through the use of cooking utensils, deodorants, and other products containing aluminum could cause the disease. A recent study of more than 1,900 people showed that cognitive decline was greater in those with a higher daily intake of aluminum from drinking water, although not all studies have confirmed this connection. It's possible that rather than causing the damage, aluminum collects in brain areas after the damage has occurred.

For optimum brain and body health, we do need a small amount of omega-6 fats in our diet—they support healthy skin and normal blood clotting. The problem is that they taste so good that we tend to eat too much. The imbalance of high levels of omega-6 relative to omega-3 fats can contribute to brain health problems. The ratio of omega-6 fats ingested versus omega-3 fats in a typical American diet is 20 to 1, but we should strive for a ratio closer to 3 to 1.

## Proteins: Getting to the Meat of It

The Alzheimer's prevention diet combines healthy nutrition from a variety of food groups, and protein is an essential component. In their study of food combinations and Alzheimer's risk, Columbia University researchers found that diets emphasizing proteins from fish and nuts in combination with generous portions of fruits and vegetables can lower the risk for Alzheimer's disease compared with diets combining red meat and butter and lower amounts of fruits and vegetables.

**TRY THIS!**

Bake two apples with a little brown sugar, cinnamon, and raisins in ½ cup of water at 400 degrees F for half an hour. You'll have a delicious dessert with under a gram of fat in it.

Eating a carbohydrate snack—perhaps an apple or a bag of pretzels—makes us feel satisfied for a while, but soon afterward we tend to feel hungry again. Adding a protein to this snack, perhaps a cup of nonfat yogurt, will provide longer-lasting appetite satisfaction, so we can better control hunger and body weight.

Amino acids are the building blocks of all proteins, which also provide the structure for the body's enzymes that maintain normal cellular function. Nine of the 20 amino acids that our bodies need are *essential* amino acids. We call them essential because the body cannot synthesize them, or make them on its own: We can only get them through our diet. Fish, poultry, meat, eggs, milk, yogurt, cheese, and soybeans all contain these nine essential amino acids.

Fish is not only a great source of omega-3 fats but it also provides healthy protein. The American Heart Association recommends eating fish twice a week. Wild salmon, halibut, light tuna, cod, flounder, sole, sea bass, shrimp, lobster, scallops, and crab are all healthy choices. Keep in mind that farmed fish has more total fat and a higher proportion of omega-6 fat than fish caught in the wild. Also, eating too much fish can increase mercury levels in the blood. Larger predatory fish such as shark and swordfish contain proportionately more mercury than smaller fish like salmon or sole.

What if you don't like fish? White meat chicken and lean beef make healthy entrée choices too, but you should give fish another try.

## Eat Brain-Friendly Carbohydrates

Compared with the rest of the body, our brains require a considerable amount of energy, and carbohydrates provide a major source of that energy. Whole-grain and high-fiber foods are brain healthy and help control weight, lower blood pressure, prevent strokes, and reduce the risk for diabetes and heart disease. The body takes longer to digest whole grains and high-fiber foods than processed foods. Examples of whole grains include 100 percent whole-grain bread, brown rice, oatmeal, and even popcorn. Eating whole grains and fresh fruits helps people feel fuller while eating fewer calories.

In processed foods, some of the vitamins, minerals, and phytonutrients have been removed. Food processing also removes the fiber from carbohydrates, which increases the food's glycemic index, or GI, the measure of how fast blood sugar rises after eating.

Carbohydrates are made up of sugar, or

### HEALTHY PROTEIN OPTIONS

**beef:** lean cuts

**chicken breast**

**cheese:** low-fat or nonfat cottage, cream (light), goat, mozzarella, ricotta, low-fat Swiss

**eggs, egg whites**

**fish:** anchovy, halibut, herring, salmon, sea bass, trout, tuna, whitefish

**milk:** low-fat or nonfat (skim)

**nuts:** almonds, walnuts; peanuts (actually legumes)

**nut butter:** almond

**soy proteins:** tofu, edamame

**turkey breast**

**yogurt:** low-fat or nonfat

glucose, and after digesting a meal, the glucose is transported from the digestive tract to the blood. The glycemic index (ranging from 0 to 100) classifies carbohydrates according to how quickly they raise blood sugar levels.

Most processed foods, including sugared cereals, cookies, crackers, and instant foods, have high GI ratings. Because they are digested and absorbed rapidly, these high-GI foods spike blood sugar levels quickly. Foods with low GI ratings, such as vegetables, fresh fruits, nonfat plain yogurt, soybeans, and nuts, are digested slowly, resulting in a slower blood sugar rise, which is healthier and keeps us satisfied longer. Research suggests that a low GI diet may decrease the risk for developing diabetes.

Investigators from the Cooper Institute in Dallas, Texas, studied more than 10,000 volunteers and found that a low glycemic diet can reduce the risk for metabolic syndrome. That's good news for brain health because metabolic syndrome increases the risk for heart disease, diabetes, and Alzheimer's disease.

# Raise a Glass for Your Brain

All my friends know that I am a lightweight when it comes to drinking alcohol. It takes only one or two glasses of wine to get me tipsy. One of my college roommates speculated that I might have some type of antisocial disease that made me allergic to alcohol. It turns out that my affliction may have been protecting my brain from Alzheimer's all along.

For years we've known about the association between drinking alcohol in moderation and having a lower risk for developing Alzheimer's disease. A recent study that included nearly 15,000 participants found that light drinkers had a nearly 30 percent lower risk for dementia when compared to people who either abstain completely or who overindulge. This was not a double-blind placebo controlled study, so it is not absolute proof that moderate drinking protects the brain, but it is still nice to know that while enjoying a glass of wine at dinner, there's a possibility that it may be protecting my brain.

Too much alcohol, however, is harmful to the brain, and just how much is too much varies according to the particular study. Some studies suggest that one glass of wine or spirits is brain protective for women and two glasses are the healthy brain limit for men. That difference between men and women may reflect the fact that men are usually larger than women and can tolerate more alcohol.

**TRY THIS!**
Set a timer for one minute and see if you can write down 20 antioxidant fruits. No cheating by going back to the list on page 97.

Some experts suggest that light alcohol consumption lowers the risk for Alzheimer's because of lifestyle factors. People who drink in moderation may deal with most aspects of their lives in moderation, and that personality style might protect their brains from chronic stress.

Another possibility is that a chemical in the alcoholic beverage protects the brain. Scientists at Mount Sinai School of Medicine, in New York, studied the effects of wine on experimental laboratory mice that possessed a human Alzheimer's gene. They found that when the mice ingested moderate amounts of cabernet sauvignon wine—the mouse equivalent of a six-ounce glass—the animals had better memory ability and less of the protein that forms the building blocks of amyloid plaques in the brain. The wine used in the study was generated using cabernet sauvignon grapes from Fresno, California. Of course, there were some mice that would have preferred French cabernets, but they had to make do with Fresno for this study.

Wine, beer, and hard liquor all appear to lower risk for Alzheimer's disease, and apparently the antioxidant chemicals in any of these forms of alcohol could be brain protective. Wine drinkers may benefit from an additional healthy brain compound found in grapes called resveratrol, which increases life span in animals in a way that is similar to caloric restriction. Some researchers believe that one might have to consume too much wine to reap the healthy brain benefits of resveratrol, but the exact amount is not known. Scientists have been trying to squeeze this ingredient out of the wine bottle and into a capsule so we all can live longer and better by popping resveratrol capsules, which are available now. It is not yet clear whether you can get the needed ingredient to reach the brain in capsule form, so all you wine lovers will be happy to know that you may still need to wash down your resveratrol capsules with a nice glass of Bordeaux.

## Caffeine: A Cup a Day May Keep Dementia Away

Some mornings Gigi gets up, grinds the coffee, and starts it brewing. The wonderful aroma of the fresh brew fills the house and I keep my eyes closed tightly until she brings me my coffee in bed along with one of the newspapers. Pure bliss.

Moderate drinking of caffeinated beverages is another way to protect your brain. A large-scale epidemiological study from Sweden reported that drinking up to three cups of coffee a day was associated with a 65 percent lower rate of developing Alzheimer's disease. A daily dose of coffee also lowers the risk for Parkinson's disease and diabetes, two age-related conditions that increase our risk for dementia.

A cup or two of joe also appears to protect the brain from the possible harmful effects of cholesterol. University of North Carolina scientists reported that when laboratory animals were fed diets high in cholesterol they found leaks in their blood–brain barriers, the natural shields that protect the brain from blood toxins. The mice that ingested daily coffee had much sturdier blood–brain barriers, so less cholesterol got into their brains.

Short-term mental effects of caffeine can be both positive and negative. Caffeine makes us more alert, increases attention, and elevates mood. Studies of learning and recall demonstrate short-term improvements following coffee consumption. But too much caffeine can make us irritable and anxious and lead to insomnia, especially when we drink it in the evening. And if you drink coffee every day, you're likely to experience caffeine withdrawal if you go without. As many of us know, the headache and lethargy from caffeine withdrawal is quite unpleasant. Keep in mind that caffeine is present in many foods and beverages. A six-ounce cup of brewed coffee contains 100 milligrams; a carbonated cola has 45 milligrams, a cup of tea has 40 milligrams, and a chocolate bar has about 10 milligrams. People who are particularly sensitive to caffeine should know that even an after-lunch espresso can have a disruptive effect on sleep later in the night. Also, as we age we become more sensitive to the effects of caffeine, and some people like to switch to decaf in the afternoon so they can still enjoy the flavor without the side effects.

## Spice It Up

Spices and herbs add color and flavoring to our foods. Although only small amounts are generally used in cooking and seasoning, they add potential health benefits from their antioxidant and other effects. For example, consuming garlic lowers cholesterol levels and blood pressure. Ginger may lessen pain in patients with arthritis, and several herbs and spices are believed to have cancer-fighting properties.

The table on page 106 illustrates the strong antioxidant potencies of several herbs and spices measured in quantities of half an ounce. All these spices provide antioxidant benefits, even in single-recipe amounts, so it's a good idea to vary your spices rather than emphasize any particular one.

Scientists recently studied piperine, the main active antioxidant ingredient in black pepper. After just two weeks, the piperine not only improved memory performance in experimental mice that carried an Alzheimer's gene, but also delayed neurodegeneration in the hippocampus memory center of their brains.

Q: I've been overweight most of my life and finally saw a nutritionist who helped me lose 30 pounds in a year. I've noticed a big improvement in my memory. Is there a connection?

A: Clinical researchers studied 150 volunteers who underwent weight-loss surgery. They found that 12 weeks after the procedure the volunteers showed significantly better memory, concentration, and problem-solving abilities. Other studies have found that a low-fat and low-carb diet improves mood as well as cognitive abilities after a year.

## Indian Food for Thought

Gigi and I love Indian food, and we have a favorite little Indian restaurant where we eat every couple of weeks. Unlike the other diners, who may be discussing their workday or plans for the weekend, we usually spar over the last piece of chicken curry while talking about how good this food is for our brains.

In the spice table at left, ground turmeric, cumin seed, and curry powder all had high scores in ORAC units for antioxidant potency. For thousands of years, curcumin has been extracted from turmeric, which is used to make spices (curry, mustard), food coloring, and medicine to treat a variety of ailments.

In part because of relatively lower rates of dementia in India compared with other countries, scientists wondered if eating curried foods might protect the brain from Alzheimer's disease. My UCLA colleagues Drs. Greg Cole and Sally Frautschy have demonstrated curcumin's potent antioxidant, anti-inflammatory, and antiamyloid properties—all effects that we'd expect to protect the brain from Alzheimer's disease. In one study of more than 1,000 volunteers between ages 60 and 93, those who ate curried foods more frequently had higher scores on standard memory tests.

### EXAMPLES OF ANTIOXIDANT SPICES

| SPICE | ANTIOXIDANT POTENCY ORAC Units per ½ Ounce |
|---|---|
| oregano, dried | 25,000 |
| cinnamon, ground | 18,800 |
| turmeric, ground | 18,200 |
| vanilla bean, dried | 17,500 |
| parsley, dried | 10,500 |
| basil, dried | 8,700 |
| cumin seed | 7,700 |
| curry powder | 6,900 |
| ginger, ground | 5,600 |
| pepper, black | 4,900 |
| chili powder | 3,400 |

Many experts believe that the oils used to cook the curried dishes help get the brain-protective ingredients into your neurons. Some people take curcumin supplements, but it is not clear whether the curcumin from supplements actually gets into the brain cells when it is not mixed in the oils used in the cooked Indian dishes. Some scientists argue that curcumin's anti-inflammatory properties stem from general responses that occur throughout the body, triggered in the stomach when curcumin is initially absorbed, so direct brain penetration may not be necessary. Our UCLA research group is currently studying this question and planning a trial of curcumin in people with age-related memory complaints to determine whether it can protect the brain from Alzheimer's. Curcumin is available in capsule form at health food stores, or as turmeric in the spice section at the supermarket.

## Feed Your Brain to Fight Alzheimer's

The scientific evidence is compelling: What we eat affects our mental function and may be critical to maintaining brain health and delaying the onset of Alzheimer's disease. As we continue to learn more about a balanced, nutritional approach to protecting brain health, keep in mind the following strategies for your Alzheimer's prevention diet:

- Emphasize complex carbohydrates and whole grains while avoiding processed foods and high glycemic index carbohydrates.
- Use mental power to control your appetite—daydream all you like about eating that unhealthy snack to avoid actually eating it.
- Calories count when controlling body weight, but individualize your diet plan to meet your needs. Low carbohydrate diets offer quick results, but it's usually best to combine a carbohydrate and a protein in a snack for longer-lasting satiety.
- Eating omega-3 fats from fish at least twice a week not only protects the brain from Alzheimer's but also stabilizes mood and fights off depression.
- Antioxidant fruits and vegetables are great brain foods. You can eat them fresh or dried or drink them in juice form.
- Healthy proteins from fish, poultry, lean beef, or soybeans fortify muscles, satisfy hunger, and provide essential amino acids.
- Alcohol and caffeine may protect the brain, but moderation is key—enjoy but don't overindulge.
- Generous helpings of herbs and spices are nutritious and good for the brain.

"THE MORE YOU USE
YOUR BRAIN, THE
MORE BRAIN YOU WILL
HAVE TO USE."

—GEORGE DORSEY,
AMERICAN ANTHROPOLOGIST

## CHAPTER 6

# Mental
# Workouts
# to Sharpen
# Your Mind

A FRIEND SENT ME AN E-MAIL with the subject line "New Brain Exercise." I opened the site and the instructions said it was going to test my observational skills—how well I pay attention to common, everyday experiences. Okay, I thought, no problem. The first question asked whether a standard traffic light has the green on the top or the bottom. I wasn't sure, so I guessed . . . wrong. The next question asked how many states there are in the U.S. My confidence returned. I got the next two questions right, but when the fifth question asked what six colors appear on a classic Campbell's soup can label, I decided I'd had enough fun and games and had better get back to work.

My brain game experience was typical of many people's: There's the excitement of the challenge, the frustration if you can't get it right, the boredom if it's too easy, and the triumph when you solve a tough one—especially if you actually figure it out rather than just guess the right answer. Mental workouts designed to strengthen neural circuits have become increasingly popular with baby boomers and seniors, thanks to multiple studies reporting a connection between stimulating mental activities and lower rates of developing Alzheimer's disease.

Today people have a variety of choices for working out their neurons, from brain gyms to interactive websites to hand-held electronic games. A challenge for consumers is to figure out what these different mental workouts actually do for their cognitive abilities, and to discover which forms of brain aerobics they enjoy so that their mental stimuli of choice will become habit forming.

## The Brain Can Change Itself

For many years scientists believed that brain cells or neurons could not change once they had developed into mature cells. More than a decade ago, however, that long-held tenet was dispelled thanks to a study revealing that new brain cell growth, or *neurogenesis,* can occur in adult humans. Dr. Fred Gage and colleagues at the Salk Institute for Biological Studies reported that primitive neural stem cells are able to grow into full-blown brain neurons. Our DNA controls neurogenesis by producing brain-derived neurotrophic factor, or BDNF, which appears to influence future brain health.

People who inherit a healthy form of BDNF have a lower risk for

Alzheimer's disease. Exercise can increase the size of the hippocampus, and higher BDNF blood levels are associated with exercise-induced enlargement in this important memory center of the brain. Functional MRI studies also show that BDNF gene expression influences neural activity in the brain's hippocampal memory center.

We know that young brains develop and change rapidly. Birth through adolescence is a period of extensive growth, where neural circuits continually take on different shapes and configurations, making it easier for young people to learn things such as how to speak foreign languages or play musical instruments. However, research has shown that even when people get older their brains remain malleable and responsive to training. After just seven hours of Internet search-engine training, people in their mid-60s demonstrated more extensive frontal lobe activity in brain regions that control decision-making and short-term memory. Other experiments have shown that the brain recruits fewer neurons and exerts less energy when we practice and become more efficient at a new task.

Q: **If I train my memory, will I become more intelligent?**

A: A recent study found that after successful memory training, fluid intelligence (reasoning and abstract thinking) improved.

Your brain is constantly sensitive to stimuli it receives—synaptic connections, neural circuits, and chemical transmitters actively respond to both external and internal cues. You have control over what you do with your brain from moment to moment, and what you choose to do has an impact on how much and how well your brain can absorb and retain new information.

## Can Doing Puzzles Prevent Alzheimer's?

I enjoy doing crossword puzzles in the newspaper every morning. It's fun and relaxing, and the more I do them, the better I get at solving the clues. Although there's no solid, double-blind study evidence that my puzzling will truly lower my future risk for Alzheimer's disease, I think it's great that I can use words like *élan* and *fillip* in a sentence.

Recent research has confirmed earlier studies showing a connection between mental stimulation and better brain health. Having a college education is associated with a lower future risk of developing Alzheimer's disease, and it appears that the more time we spend engaged in various stimulating mental activities, the greater the delay in mental decline. In a recent analysis involving more than 5,600 people age 65 and older, engaging in stimulating leisure activities over a four-year period resulted in significant delays in the onset of dementia and Alzheimer's disease.

These kinds of epidemiological studies linking mental stimulation to better brain health encourage me to work harder on the notorious Sunday-morning crossword, with or without absolute proof of brain protection. Animal studies provide additional evidence that mental stimulation improves brain health. Small animals that grow up in mentally stimulating cages filled with toys and other fun things end up with significantly more brain cells in their hippocampal memory centers compared with animals raised in standard-issue cages. These animal studies also show that stimulating environments lead to new brain cell growth and more synaptic connections between neurons. The animals also perform better on memory tests.

In a recent study of more than 3,000 people age 32 to 84, Dr. Margie Lachman and colleagues at Brandeis University confirmed earlier reports of an association between higher education and lower risk for Alzheimer's disease. Her team reported that the more years of education completed by the participants, the better they performed on cognitive tests assessing a range of skills, including mental flexibility, memory, complex reasoning, and abstract thinking. The investigators found that some of the people with less educational achievement also performed well on cognitive tests. These people spent more time engaged in stimulating cognitive activities (such as reading, playing Scrabble, doing crossword puzzles, attending lectures, and writing letters) than others with less formal education. Apparently, mental exercise throughout life compensates for lower educational achievement. So even if you feel that you didn't get enough formal education, continued cognitive stimulation could provide you the edge you need to kick your Ph.D. pal's butt the next time you two play Scrabble.

A few years ago a friend told me that after he heard that mentally challenging games and puzzles might improve his brain health, he had been forcing himself to do crosswords and other puzzles every day even though he didn't find them fun or challenging. I suggested that he might be better off doing other brain-stimulating things that he did enjoy, like playing chess and reading, and not worry so much about becoming a puzzle master. Besides, he had a mentally challenging job as a university professor and probably didn't need much, if any, more mental exercise in his life. He now skips the puzzle section of the newspaper and feels no guilt about it.

## The Upside of Brain Aging

Most people know that aging chips away at their short-term memory, but those same individuals may not be aware of the upside of their aging brains. Thanks to years of mental activity, our frontal lobes get better at solving complex problems and grasping the big picture of things.

At UCLA our research team was able to rapidly train people in their 60s to perform novel mental tasks like Internet searching. The training resulted in significant increases in neural activity in an area of the frontal lobe that controls working memory. This is the very short memory skill we use to hold information in mind long enough to use it quickly.

When psychologists provide specific training to improve short-term, or working, memory, it also benefits frontal lobe skills that allow research subjects to solve new problems. And the longer the training period, the greater the observed improvements, possibly explaining the better frontal lobe skills of a middle ager or senior compared to a teenager or a 20-something.

Neuroscientists have found that during midlife our neurons may be especially agile because of extra white matter build-up. White matter coats the long axons, the wires in our brains that transmit messages from one cell to another. UCLA investigators discovered that this white matter coating peaks at about 50 years of age, which may reflect the faster transmission of neural messages in midlife.

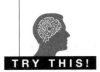

**TRY THIS!**

Create a crossword puzzle out of three words. Now add on three more words. To make it challenging, try to include the letter X, Q, or Z.

Another advantage to an older brain is that both sides—the right and left hemispheres—communicate more effectively than they do in a younger brain. Brain scan studies show that older study subjects have nearly equal levels of activity when performing memory tests or problem-solving tasks, whereas younger volunteers tend to favor either the right or left side of the brain when performing the same tasks. Duke University scientists found that mentally successful seniors are more likely to use both hemispheres together when performing cognitive tasks. The more effective older brain that uses both hemispheres in unison may compensate for age-related declines, just as we are better off lifting a heavy weight with both hands than just one.

## Hanging Out with Friends Protects Your Brain

Humans are social animals. Nearly all of us enjoy a stimulating conversation or a friendly debate. Discussions often get us thinking about new ideas and make us want to learn more.

A recent study affirms my impression that social interactions boost cognitive ability. Dr. Oscar Ybarra and associates studied the immediate cognitive effects of a stimulating ten-minute conversation about privacy protection in light of new technologies and political events. The investigators found that after these brief discussions, the study subjects had better and quicker short-term memory abilities than did a control group. The study's control group engaged in a more passive social interaction: watching a ten-minute clip of the sitcom *Seinfeld*. Despite these findings, I refuse to give up watching *Seinfeld* reruns—I'm convinced that they protect my brain by lowering my stress level.

Interacting with other people also helps us avoid feelings of loneliness, which can protect brain health because associating with others appears to decrease our risk for Alzheimer's disease, even if we like being alone. Dr. Steven Cole and associates at UCLA discovered a possible connection between loneliness and dementia risk. They found that chronically lonely people overexpress genes linked to inflammation, which can cause brain cell damage and neural degeneration. The good news is that becoming and staying socially engaged may reduce your risk for dementia by as much as 60 percent.

The brain protective effects of social interactions may stem from several benefits of the company of others. When we talk with friends about our concerns, their empathic responses may lessen our worries and stress levels. Hanging out with people who embrace a healthy lifestyle can also encourage us to stick with our own Alzheimer's prevention routine—good habits can be contagious. The cognitive exercise of keeping up with a conversation also appears to stimulate and possibly protect our neurons.

## Cross Train Your Brain

Our brains crave variety. When we notice or experience something new, it perks up our attention and usually brings us pleasure. Unfamiliar stimuli and new mental challenges stimulate neuronal growth in the brain's reticular formation, a region that may have developed novelty-seeking specialization as a survival mechanism to improve our ancestors' ability to detect predators.

Our UCLA research shows that engaging in mental activities increases neural activation and communication throughout the brain. This kind of brain cross talk might offer another form of neural protection. Psychologist Ellen Bialystok and associates in Toronto, Canada, found that people who speak more than one language avoided Alzheimer's disease for a longer period than study subjects who only spoke one language. The findings are consistent with the idea that bilingual individuals have to work the brain's executive control networks more often, constantly deciding which of their two languages to use. This process of sorting through multiple options appears to strengthen neurons.

We know that as the brain matures, the right and left hemispheres work together more effectively, but these two sides of the brain still maintain considerable specialization throughout life. For the average right-handed individual, the *left hemisphere* is more analytical and verbal and controls the following functions:

- logical thinking and reasoning
- sequencing information, making lists, and organizing thoughts
- speech and language
- counting and mathematics
- recognizing symbols
- reading and writing

For that same average person, the *right hemisphere* is more visual and emotional and controls the following functions:

- spatial relationships like reading maps
- musical and artistic talents
- recognizing faces
- perceiving depth
- sense of humor
- expressing and reading emotions

For people who are left-handed, the left hemisphere is the visual and emotional brain, while the right hemisphere is the analytical and verbal brain.

Brain scan studies show that we can build brain muscle specific to the hemisphere we are working out. London taxi drivers have larger hippocampal memory centers in the right hemisphere, the side of the brain that controls visual-spatial skills. Years of reading and memorizing maps has built up the brain bulk in the regions that control those abilities. Separate studies of jugglers show that it doesn't take years to build the right side of the brain—it can occur in just months. Functional MRI studies also demonstrate increased left-hemisphere activation during speech and language tasks.

Ideally, you will want to work both hemispheres, and you may want to alternate your mental aerobic stimulation program from the left hemisphere to the right hemisphere and back again. Because the brain likes variety, cross training the brain makes sense. Fitness trainers often cross train, or vary workouts, at the gym to build stamina in different muscle groups and avoid repeating the same exercise routine day after day. In a similar way, cross training the brain will challenge mental athletes, minimize their boredom, and optimize cognitive results.

## Computer Games to Aerobicize Your Mind

With the intriguing findings on how brain exercise may do more than boost Sudoku puzzle skills, the brain fitness software business has been growing at a rate of about 50 percent every year. Some experts estimate that by 2015 the brain fitness market will reach $2 billion annually.

These games are available online and off-line and come in all shapes and sizes (see Appendix 2). One game may improve driving skills, and a large insurance company has distributed the program to older drivers in Pennsylvania to determine its effectiveness in reducing car accidents. Another company has developed a touch-screen device to engage seniors with film clips, images, and music from their youth. It is the most popular brain game in assisted living facilities throughout the U.S.

Despite considerable growth, this new industry has received mixed reviews. The challenge for game developers is to come up with programs that not only offer a fun and engaging experience but also provide cognitive benefits. Some critics are skeptical that the skills derived from these games truly transfer a benefit to everyday cognitive tasks.

The debate was recently fueled by a study published in the journal *Nature*, which reported the results of a six-week, online cognitive training course. More than 11,000 participants trained on several games a week using cognitive tasks designed to improve reasoning, memory, visual-spatial skills, planning, and attention. Although training improved the cognitive skills needed to play the games, the investigators couldn't detect benefits that improved daily function.

Where some brain games fall short is in explicitly teaching gamers how to transfer the cognitive skills they pick up in the game to their everyday life situations. Our UCLA group found that when we guided people on how to apply their new cognitive techniques to everyday memory challenges, they were able to enjoy the practical benefits of their training. Both our off-line and online courses emphasize this approach, as do the memory techniques introduced in Chapters 3 and 9 as part of the Alzheimer's prevention program.

It's also important to distinguish between targeted cognitive skill training that teaches specific memory techniques, and mental aerobics that exercise a range of mental abilities. The latter exercises are a way to challenge our minds and strengthen our neurons while having fun.

## Awaken Sleepy Neurons

For as long as I can remember, I've heard that we use only 20 percent of our brain power. That is a myth. However, some areas of the brain do not get used as much as others, and we should directly stimulate brain regions that have been at rest in order to keep them limber and awake, ready to process new stimuli.

Our brains pass information through billions of dendrites, or neural extensions, like tree branches that grow smaller as they extend outward. When we don't use our dendrites, they can shrink or atrophy, but waking them up with mental exercise reactivates their connections to pass novel information along. New dendrites can be created after old ones die.

Brain games aim to stimulate our minds and work out our dendrites so they extend their branches. The point is to challenge our brains and strengthen our brain cell connections. The fun factor of puzzles and brain teasers comes from pushing ourselves to make a mental leap beyond our usual assumptions. It's exciting to find new solutions to what appear to be either too easy or impossible problems. Of course, not everyone likes brain teasers and puzzles. Don't fret if you'd prefer to read a novel or take a nature walk instead. Although doing mental aerobics may wake up your neurons and do them some good, if you don't find them fun and engaging, move on to other activities that you do enjoy.

Our first impression of a visual image often remains fixed in our mind unless we make a conscious effort to perceive an alternate interpretation, as in the simple image of a book below:

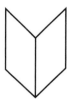

Does your brain initially perceive the cover pointing toward you? Can you push your dendrites to flip it around and see the open book facing you?

Sometimes this kind of flip-flopping of neuronal circuits can be fun. Other times it can be mind-boggling, as in many M.C. Escher drawings or in the following optical illusion:

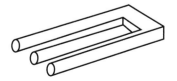

As you awaken your neuronal networks, you'll find that you can build up your creative thinking skills. You will be stimulating and strengthening your neurons, bolstering healthy dendrites, and extending their branches to make new connections.

## Brain Games Sampler

The brain teasers that follow will give you a sample of the kinds of exercises you can do to tweak your neural circuits. You don't have to enroll in an intensive course of conversational French or begin a marathon of power Scrabble to build brain muscle. The key is to discover new challenging mental activities that you also enjoy so that you will want to continue them over time. Perhaps you love pop music but are curious about the symphony. Go check it out. Or maybe you've always loved piano recitals but have never taken a lesson. Try it—you might enjoy it.

The key is to train but not strain your brain. To help you find your mental aerobics sweet spot, I have included a range of exercises from beginning to advanced. They are arranged to cross train your brain, jumping from right-brain to left-brain workouts. Once you figure out what type of brain games you enjoy, you may wish to check the Internet or other resources to keep shaking up your mental challenges.

---

**BEGINNING EXERCISES** (Answers on p. 124)

1. WARMING UP. I like to stretch a little in the morning before I do my physical workout. Engaging neural circuits in ways that are different from their usual patterns provides a good mental stretch and warm up.

   Try this one: Take a piece of paper and a pencil and use your non-dominant hand (i.e., left hand if you are right-handed) to write your first and last name in cursive.

2. LETTER SCRAMBLE. This puzzle will tweak your left-brain language centers and your frontal lobe.

From the scrambled letters below, see how many words of three or more letters you can write down. For extra credit, set your timer for four minutes. Ready, set, go:

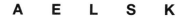

**A   E   L   S   K**

\_\_\_\_  \_\_\_\_  \_\_\_\_  \_\_\_\_  \_\_\_\_

3. COUNTING SQUARES. Let's get your right brain charged up with your frontal lobe in the visual spatial puzzle below.

Count up the number of squares in the figure to the right.

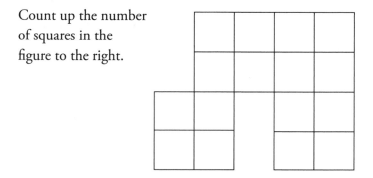

4. HIDDEN PROVERB. Proverbs exercise abstract thinking. Here's a twist on a familiar proverb.

The vowels have been removed, and the remaining letters broken up into groups of two or three letters each. Replace the vowels and find the proverb:

**PNN   YFR   YR   THG   HTS**

_____

_____

5. ROTATING FIGURES. Here's a right-brainer that works your ability to rotate images.

Look at the object on the left and then choose the version that matches (A, B, or C).

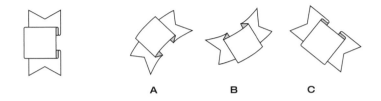

6. WORDPLAY. Here's more brain fun with letters and words.

Beginning with the word HAND, change one letter at a time until you come up with the word CART. Each change must spell another word.

**H  A  N  D**

—  —  —  —

—  —  —  —

**C  A  R  T**

There may be several correct answers.

7. ROTATING FIGURES IN SEQUENCE. This exercise requires you to pick out the sequence and rotate images at the same time. Give it a try to pump up your right hemisphere.

Complete the sequence by choosing object A, B, or C:

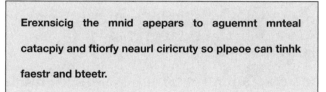

8. SPELL CHECK. As our brains age, we are often able to recognize patterns and derive meaning from words, even when those words are misspelled and appear to be gibberish.

See how well you do with the sentence in the box below:

> **Erexnsicig the mnid apepars to aguemnt mnteal catacpiy and ftiorfy neaurl ciricruty so plpeoe can tinhk faestr and bteetr.**

9. GROUP SORTING. Picking out patterns often involves figuring out whether an item belongs to a particular group. Practice your pattern recognition skills with the items below.

You'll note three types of items. Try to quickly sort them into groups. Set your timer for 30 seconds:

| | | |
|---|---|---|
| ruler | clipper | colander |
| spatula | rake | mower |
| eraser | scissor | pot |
| whisk | pencil | hoe |

10. WORD RECOGNITION. Figure out the one word suggested by the three words in the box below.

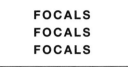

## ANSWERS TO BEGINNING EXERCISES

1. WARMING UP. No right answer.

2. LETTER SCRAMBLE. Here are the words I wrote down. You may have found others as well:
ALE, ALES, ASK
ELK, ELKS, ELS
KALE
LAS, LAKE, LAKES, LEA, LEAS, LEAK, LEAKS
SAKE, SALE, SEA, SEAL

3. COUNTING SQUARES. 22 (don't forget all the combinations of squares within squares).

4. HIDDEN PROVERB. A PENNY FOR YOUR THOUGHTS.

5. ROTATING FIGURES. C

6. WORD PLAY. Here's my solution to the puzzle (changed letters are bold and underlined):

HAND
HA**R**D
**C**ARD
CAR**T**

7. ROTATING FIGURES IN SEQUENCE. B

8. SPELL CHECK.

> Exercising the mind appears to augment mental capacity and fortify neural circuitry so people can think faster and better.

9. GROUP SORTING.
Office supplies: ruler, scissors, pencil, eraser
Cooking utensils: spatula, colander, pot, whisk
Gardening tools: clipper, rake, mower, hoe

10. WORD RECOGNITION. Trifocals

If you enjoyed these mental challenges and didn't get too frustrated, consider moving on to the intermediate exercises that follow. Otherwise, repeat these exercises tomorrow and perhaps check out some websites and puzzle books with brainteasers at a similar level of difficulty before ratcheting up to harder puzzles. The next group of puzzles is a bit more challenging, but can be even more fun.

**INTERMEDIATE EXERCISES (Answers on p. 129)**

1. CURSIVE ON THE LEFT. Take your nondominant handwriting exercise to the next level:

   Use a piece of paper and a pencil with your nondominant hand (i.e., left hand if you are right-handed) to write your first and last name in cursive, and then write it backward. Good luck.

2. LETTER SCRAMBLE SEQUEL. Here's a fresh batch of scrambled letters. See how many words of three letters or more you can write down this time. To make the exercise a bit tougher, set your timer for three minutes.

## T R E I O A

3. FLIP THE GOALPOST. Here's a stimulating teaser that uses only four toothpicks or matchsticks, but will score points for your frontal lobe.

   Arrange the toothpicks in the shape of a football goalpost as shown below. By moving only two of the toothpicks, see if you can reverse the direction of the goalpost (make it go upside down).

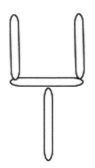

4. ANOTHER HIDDEN PROVERB. Expand your abstract thinking with this exercise.

All the vowels have have been taken out of the following proverb, and the remaining letters are broken up into groups of three to five letters each. Replace the vowels and find the proverb:

**B R D N     T H H     N D S**

**W R T     H T W N     T H B S H**

5. BODY PARTS. Here is a challenging brainteaser that will activate those neurons in your prefrontal cortex:

Name the ten body parts that have only three letters. The T word for breast and the A word for buttocks don't count.

6. WORD GRID POWER. Here's one that will draw out both your visual spatial skills and your verbal skills.

Use the letters I I L D N N A A E E S S to complete the following grid, which will need to spell out words that read the same across as down.

| | | | P |
|---|---|---|---|
| | | E | |
| | E | | |
| P | | | |

7. NUMBERING OFFICES. This riddle will give you a chance to let your logical and mathematical skills shine.

Gloria's job is to hang the numbers on all the doors of the second floor of a new downtown office building, which includes suites

200 to 299. How many of the number 2 will she need to complete her assignment?

8. JUMBLED LETTERS. Let's awaken your word power skills with this teaser. Take your time and concentrate, and you should get the right answer.

See if you can find the letters mixed up below that spell the names of two brain-healthy spices. Use each letter only once.

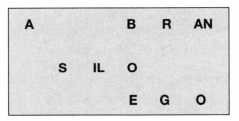

9. TAKE A HINT. Figure out the message suggested by the word in the box below.

10. REVERSE GEOGRAPHY. Which of the following does not belong in the set?

**K R O Y     W E N     N A G I H C I M**

**A W O I     A N A I D N I     O I H O**

**S I O N I L L I     A T O S E N N I M**

## ANSWERS TO INTERMEDIATE EXERCISES

1. **CURSIVE ON THE LEFT.** No right answer.

2. **LETTER SCRAMBLE.** Here are the words I wrote down. You may have found others as well:

   TAR, TARE, TEAR, TIE, TIER, TIRE, TOE, TOR, TORE, TRIO
   RAT, RATE, RITE, ROT
   EAT, EAR
   IOTA, IRATE, IRE
   OAR, OAT, ORATE, ORE
   ART, ATE

3. **FLIP THE GOALPOST.** Slide the horizontal toothpick to the left until the left upper vertical toothpick touches its center. Then bring down the right upper vertical toothpick that's left on its own, so that its upper point touches the left point of the horizontal toothpick. Or do the converse: Move the horizontal toothpick to the right as described, then move the left upper vertical toothpick down. You now have an upside down goalpost with just two moves.

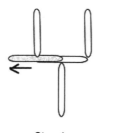 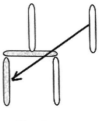

**Step 1**            **Step 2**

4. **HIDDEN PROVERB.**
   A BIRD IN THE HAND IS WORTH TWO IN THE BUSH.

5. **BODY PARTS.**
   ARM, EAR, EYE, GUM, HIP, JAW, LEG, LIP, RIB, TOE

6. WORD GRID POWER.

| L | I | S | P |
|---|---|---|---|
| I | D | E | A |
| S | E | E | N |
| P | A | N | E |

7. NUMBERING OFFICES. She will need 120 of the number 2. Remember, she'll need an extra 2 for 220–229 as well as the other 2s that she'll need.

8. JUMBLED LETTERS. Oregano and basil.

9. TAKE A HINT. Hurry up.

10. REVERSE GEOGRAPHY. "AWOI" is the one that does not belong. The seven words are seven U.S. states spelled backward, and Iowa is the only one of those states that does not border a Great Lake. A second correct answer is "KROY WEN" since New York is the only non-Midwestern state in the group.

Assuming you are not completely burned out from all this mental lifting, you may want to move on to the advanced exercises.

**ADVANCED EXERCISES** (Answers on p. 133)

1. **THREE-DIMENSIONAL DRAWING.** Let's tweak your brain hemispheres once again by taking out a piece of paper and drawing the following three-dimensional image with your non-dominant hand:

2. **HIDDEN WORDS.** The jumbled letters below can be rearranged

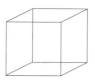

to spell out an antioxidant fruit. See if you can find it.

### Y E R     Y S E     B N     B R O

3. **WHICH SWITCH WORKS?** Here's an old mental twister that never ceases to amuse some of us puzzle fanatics and can give your frontal lobe a good workout:

A lightbulb is hanging in a room, and outside the room there are three switches. Only one of the switches connects to the bulb. All three switches are in the off position and the bulb is not lit. If you can only go in the room once to see if the bulb is lit or not (the bulb cannot be seen from outside), how can you determine which of the three switches will turn on the bulb?

4. **WORLD GEOGRAPHY.** See if you can stretch your frontal lobe again and come up with the ten countries whose name is composed of only four letters.

5. **MISSING LETTERS.** Fill in the two missing letters and unscramble the letters to find the famous English naturalist whose theory had a major impact on 20th-century thinking. Use

each letter only once.

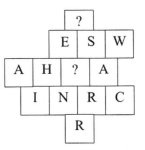

6. MORE TOOTHPICK FUN. Arrange 12 toothpicks as displayed below, and then try to create three triangles by moving only four of the toothpicks.

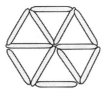

7. TRICKY EQUATION. The following equation is incorrect. How can you make it correct without moving a single line?

$$X + | \ = | X$$

8. THINKING INSIDE THE BOX. What is implied by the word in the box below?

S
T
O N E

MENTAL WORKOUTS TO SHARPEN YOUR MIND

9. NUMBER SEQUENCE. Figure out the next number in the sequence below:

**2   7   4   1   4   6   2   1   8   2**

10. ASKING FOR DIRECTIONS. You need directions to the museum because you are a bit lost. You finally get to the street you were looking for, but are not sure whether to turn left or right. You recognize two acquaintances from work, Stuart and Maurice, and decide to ask them for directions. You don't know them well but recall that one of them always tells the truth while the other always lies—you just can't remember which one is the liar and which one is the truth teller. How can you find out which way to turn by asking only one of them one question?

## ANSWERS TO ADVANCED EXERCISES

1. THREE-DIMENSIONAL DRAWING. No right answer.

2. HIDDEN WORDS. Boysenberry.

3. WHICH SWITCH WORKS? To find the correct switch (1, 2, or 3), turn switch 1 to the on position and leave it there for a few minutes. Then turn switch 1 back to the off position and turn switch 2 to the on position and enter the room. If the lightbulb is lit, then switch 2 is connected to it. If it is not lit, then either switch 1 or 3 is connected to the bulb. Briefly touch the bulb to determine which one. If the bulb is still hot, switch 1 is the correct answer; if the bulb is cold, switch 3 is connected to the bulb.

4. WORLD GEOGRAPHY.

Chad, Cuba, Fiji, Iran, Iraq, Laos, Mali, Oman, Peru, Togo

5. MISSING LETTERS. CHARLES DARWIN (L and D are the missing letters).

6. MORE TOOTHPICK FUN.

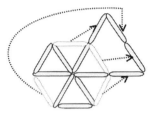

7. TRICKY EQUATION. Turn the book upside down—you'll see 11, 1, and 10 in roman numerals.

8. THINKING INSIDE THE BOX. Cornerstone.

9. NUMBER SEQUENCE. The sequence actually includes two different sequences that are interspersed. The first sequence is 2-4-6-8- . . . and the second sequence is 7-14-21-28- . . . The correct answer is: 8.

10. ASKING FOR DIRECTIONS. You should ask Stuart, "If I turn left, will I find the museum according to Maurice?" If Stuart answers yes, then you should turn right; if he answers no, then you should turn left.

    Here is the explanation: If Stuart tells the truth, Maurice is always lying, so you need to do the opposite of whatever Stuart tells you (he will be telling Maurice's lie and incorrect directions). Conversely, if Stuart is a liar, he will always be telling you the opposite of the true directions that Maurice is providing.

# Keep Building Your Brain Muscle

Most experts recommend that people remain mentally engaged and stimulated throughout life. A recent study from investigators at University College in London suggest that people who delay retirement by several years have better cognitive abilities than those who retire earlier. Whether mental workouts definitely stave off Alzheimer's disease symptoms still requires extensive, long-term prospective studies. Still, it's fun to exercise our brains, and it can improve the quality of our lives. While we wait for results from definitive studies, keep in mind some of these important points:

- Our brains are sensitive to stimuli from moment to moment. Mental stimulation appears to strengthen specific synaptic connections and neural circuits, most likely protecting our brains from Alzheimer's disease.

- Brain aging is not all bad—our neural circuitry fires faster and our frontal lobes work better as we age, allowing us to grasp the big picture and solve complex problems more rapidly.

- Staying socially connected improves our cognitive abilities and lowers our risk for Alzheimer's disease, so try to hang out with friends whenever you can, especially those who can keep you engaged in a good conversation.

- Our brains crave variety, so try to diversify your mental workouts to cross train your right and left brain hemispheres.

- Try balancing your off-line brain games with online cognitive training to see if you enjoy and benefit from this sometimes convenient and effective alternative approach.

Q: How do games and puzzles affect my brain health, and what is the best brain game for a mental workout?

A: We know that we can alter brain neural circuitry and create greater mental efficiency by playing brain games. Large epidemiological studies have found an association between spending more time doing puzzles or reading and a lower risk for developing Alzheimer's disease; however, studies demonstrating absolute proof of a cause-and-effect relationship have not been completed. Rather than wait decades for the culmination of these studies, most experts recommend that people enjoy their brain games but not count on them alone to alter their brain health. The best games for any individual are the ones they find challenging and enjoy the most. Also, because our brains are drawn to variety, varying your games is a good approach to consider.

"REALITY IS THE
LEADING CAUSE OF
STRESS FOR THOSE IN
TOUCH WITH IT."

—JANE WAGNER,
AMERICAN PLAYWRIGHT

## CHAPTER 7

# Reduce Stress

# to Fortify

# Neurons

S YLVIA M., A 44-YEAR-OLD TEACHER, became anxious about her memory changes when her mother was diagnosed with Alzheimer's disease at age 72. It was only three years since her maternal uncle had died at 75 with some type of dementia. Sylvia didn't want to get tested for Alzheimer's genes—she just wanted to start doing whatever she could to protect her brain from the disease for as long as possible.

She read everything she could get her hands on about brain health and preventing Alzheimer's. But as a single parent, caring for her two kids and now her mother, Sylvia found little time to exercise, do crossword puzzles, or eat a healthy diet and still keep up with her work. She also worried that all her multitasking and chronic stress was wreaking havoc on her memory. She was constantly misplacing things and forgetting details. And though she felt as though she was the only one stepping up and doing anything for her mom, she was reluctant to ask her younger sister and brother for help. Besides, they were both preoccupied with their own lives.

Despite her frenetic schedule, she managed to squeeze in a couple of weeks of yoga, jogging, and weight-lifting before throwing out her back. Now she had to fit physical therapy into her schedule as well. Sylvia got so overwhelmed that she forgot twice to take home the papers she was supposed to grade. She was convinced that this was the first sign of Alzheimer's eating away at her brain. Sylvia also started having trouble sleeping and lost her appetite. When she finally dragged herself into my office, it was clear that she was anxious and depressed.

What Sylvia's Alzheimer's prevention program lacked was a realistic way to manage her stress. Apparently her twice-weekly yoga classes weren't enough. I helped her understand that her fear of Alzheimer's disease coupled with her anxiety about her job and caring for her mother and kids was actually worsening her memory and possibly even raising her risk for developing dementia. I prescribed a sedating antidepressant that helped her mood and her sleep. She worried less, became more focused, and her memory improved. Eventually she became more confident about asking others for help, and once her sister and brother got involved in their mother's care, Sylvia felt less alone.

Nearly everyone faces some stress in their life. Much of Sylvia's came from her concern about a family risk for Alzheimer's disease and what would happen to her kids if she got it. She began interpreting every middle-aged memory slip as the first sign of the disease taking over her brain.

She didn't realize that her depression was adding to her memory lapses—in part brought on by her feelings of loss about her mother, as well as her other worries. Caregivers of patients with dementia have a high risk for getting depressed—some studies indicate that at least 50 percent of caregivers develop depression that requires medical treatment.

Sylvia's current memory slips probably had nothing to do with her family history of Alzheimer's. When a genetic risk contributes to Alzheimer's disease in a family, it usually strikes relatives at around the same age. Sylvia's relatives developed symptoms in their seventies. If Sylvia did have a genetic risk, her symptoms probably wouldn't emerge for another 30 years.

Sylvia wasn't aware of how much she contributed to her own high level of stress. Nobody can change their genetic predisposition for Alzheimer's, but once Sylvia knew the facts about her actual risk, she became less alarmed about her everyday memory challenges. She learned new ways to manage her stress, which not only improved her brain health but made her life more enjoyable.

## Stress, Depression, and Risk for Alzheimer's

We know that stress can create havoc in our lives and contribute to a variety of physical illnesses ranging from ulcers to heart disease. It also poses a threat to brain health and increases an individual's risk for Alzheimer's disease. Dr. Lena Johansson and colleagues at the University of Gothenburg, in Sweden, assessed levels of psychological stress in more than 1,100 women between ages 38 and 60. Her research group defined stress as symptoms of nervousness, irritation, tension, anxiety, fear, or sleep problems. After following these women for 35 years, the scientists discovered that those who experienced frequent stress in midlife had a 65 percent greater risk for Alzheimer's disease compared to those who did not experience frequent stress.

Investigators at Rush University Medical Center, in Chicago, investigated whether people who got stressed out easily were at greater risk for developing Alzheimer's disease. They measured proneness to stress (a stable personality trait indicating a tendency to experience psychological discomfort) and discovered that those who were more prone to stress were twice as likely to develop Alzheimer's disease after five years compared to those who were able to cope better. The volunteers who were prone to stress were also ten times more likely to develop mild forms of age-related memory decline.

Many studies have shown that older people with symptoms of depression have a greater risk for developing memory decline, and eventually dementia, over the years. Depression has immediate effects on mental capacity as well—it slows down the pace at which people think. People with more severe symptoms of depression have greater difficulties in problem solving and carrying out everyday activities.

These studies of human volunteers are consistent with previous work done with stressed-out laboratory animals. Dr. Robert Sapolsky of Stanford University has shown that chronic stress in laboratory mice leads to *atrophy*, or shrinkage, of the hippocampus, a brain area that controls memory processing, and these animals with a smaller hippocampus have trouble finding their way through mazes. Sapolsky's group agrees with other neuroscientists that stress hormones may be damaging the brain by aggravating a chronic inflammatory response.

## This Is Your Brain on Stress

The human brain evolved over thousands of years to respond to acute stress in a way that ensured the survival of our species. Our cavemen ancestors adapted to stress with a fight-or-flight reaction, and our brains became hard-wired to respond to stress hormones that help us put aside all other thoughts and become acutely alert to imminent dangers around us so we can quickly detect threats and either counterattack or flee.

That's fine for acute stress involving life-threatening danger such as an oncoming tiger or perhaps a large group of stampeding elephants. Plus, the physiological cascade of hormones released and other events that occurred in our brains and bodies led to evolutionary success for the ancestors of our species. Nowadays, unfortunately, when our stress is caused by dangers such as the Internet going down or perhaps credit card fraud, this hard-wired acute stress response can become chronic, and those same stress hormones that are released can cause wear and tear on our neurons, worsening memory and possibly contributing to Alzheimer's disease.

Researchers at the University of Wisconsin are finding that the stress stimulated by modern threats causes a shift in the natural balance of attention in the brain, disrupting our ability to solve complex problems and think with clarity. When the brain shifts into a stress-alert mode, it must process a large amount of data by quickly scanning the environment in an attempt to detect any looming danger. This series of events creates a form of information overload that actually impairs focused attention and problem solving. Studies of electrical activity in the brain during an acute stress attack show a shift away from the brain's frontal executive centers to the amygdala, an area beneath the temples that controls a range of emotional reactions. When confronted with stress, the emotional amygdala takes over—we tend to react quickly and instinctively, with less thought, and we often have trouble making reasonable decisions. That's why it's not a good idea to make important decisions while experiencing severe stress or anxiety.

Cortisol is one of the hormones the body secretes while under stress, helping us adapt to severe threats. When released, cortisol shifts blood flow to the brain to help focus our attention. It also shifts blood from the stomach to the muscles. Our brains sense pending danger, so appetite declines and we perceive a need for our muscles to have increased energy, strength, and speed of movement.

Studies show that after several days of cortisol injections, human volunteers experience impaired verbal memory ability. They have considerable difficulty remembering details of information they have read. The good news is that these impairments are temporary. Memory ability returns once the cortisol levels revert to normal. It's interesting to note that other recent studies indicate that when we're under stress, some forms of emotional memory may actually improve, which is consistent with the research showing that the amygdala's emotional center may become more active in stressful situations.

## Stress Changes the Body and the Brain

We all react differently to triggers of stress and anxiety, and this creates a range of symptoms, both physical and psychological. Because stress affects both the body and the brain, it is helpful to determine any health issues that might be contributing to stress and their underlying causes.

When psychiatrists sort through these various symptoms, they first look for any physical illnesses or medication side effects that might be the source of the problem. Next they search for symptom clusters or particular syndromes that point to an underlying cause. For example, the cluster of insomnia, weight loss, fatigue, and poor concentration points to depression as a likely cause. When a patient complains of trembling, upset stomach, indecisiveness, tension, and worry, an anxiety or panic disorder might be the culprit. Each of these symptom clusters has different treatment approaches that have been shown to be effective in relieving the symptoms.

## SYMPTOMS OF STRESS

### PHYSICAL

aches and pains
appetite change
fatigue
cold hands and feet
fidgeting
headache
insomnia
nail-biting
pacing
rapid heart rate
sweating
trembling
upset stomach

### MENTAL

anger
anxiety
confusion
depression
fear
frustration
impatience
tension
indecisiveness
irritability
poor concentration
memory loss
poor sense of humor

## Sleep Recharges Your Brain

I love the way I feel in the morning after a good night's sleep. My body is rested; my mind feels clear and alert; and I am happy to just linger in bed and relax. Of course, this delightful state is eventually interrupted by an alarm going off or the dog barking for me to feed him.

But long after I've gotten up and fed the dog, I continue to feel good if I've slept well during the night. It's as if my entire system—my body and my brain—has been reset in a healthy way.

Part of this good feeling may result from the anti-inflammatory effect of sleep. We have seen how chronic brain inflammation appears to contribute to the cellular deterioration that can lead to Alzheimer's disease. Getting a good night's sleep has a positive impact on that inflammatory process and may explain why people who regularly sleep well feel better and have more energy.

When scientists measure a volunteer's blood markers of inflammation, they find that after the volunteer has had a restful night of sleep, those measures improve significantly. These are the same measures that improve when we eat anti-inflammatory foods such as omega-3–rich fish. Dr. Wendy Troxel and colleagues at the University of Pittsburgh have found that people with sleep problems such as difficulty falling asleep, fretful sleep, or loud snoring have a higher risk for metabolic syndrome, another condition linked to chronic inflammation that puts the brain at risk for neural degeneration.

Most of us tend to think about sleep as a very passive mental experience. In fact, our brains are extremely active during sleep. Scientific evidence tells us that actually sleeping on our problems is an efficient way to solve them. During sleep our brain's memory centers are busy working to consolidate recall for more effective memory when we're awake. Getting a good night's sleep is an important way to improve your memory ability and reduce chronic inflammation.

## GET A GOOD NIGHT'S SLEEP

About 30 percent of people suffer from insomnia. The following are a few strategies to consider if you're having trouble falling or staying asleep through the night.

STAY UP DURING THE DAY. Daytime naps can be invigorating, but if you already suffer from sleeplessness at night, try to avoid them so you'll feel more fatigued at bedtime.

AVOID EVENING LIQUIDS. After dinner, try not to drink large quantities of water or other drinks. A full bladder can awaken you during the night and you may have trouble getting back to sleep.

KEEP A LOW PROFILE IN THE EVENING. Watching lively evening sports or a movie thriller tends to hype some people up, making it harder for them to fall asleep. Even reading a good book keeps some people from falling asleep. Exercise in the evening relaxes some people, but others find it keeps them awake. Experiment with how your brain and body respond to the timing of your nightly activities.

AVOID CAFFEINE AT NIGHT. Whether it's from tea, coffee, or even a chocolate bar, caffeine can keep us awake, so avoiding it in the evenings can help us sleep more soundly. Try to skip coffee entirely in the late afternoon and evening. And remember that cola has a lot of caffeine, as well. Try herb tea, such as mint or chamomile, which has no caffeine.

SLEEP HABITS. Create a regular sleep routine that you stick to. It can help to pick the same time at night to get into bed. Once in bed, do not watch TV, eat, or even read a book—turn out the light and take a few moments to get settled. If you are not asleep after 20 minutes, get out of bed and do something until you feel tired again. Once you go back to bed, get settled and give it another 20 minutes. Every time you get into bed to sleep, try remaining still and focus on slow, steady breathing.

# The Stress of Technology and Multitasking

Valerie H., a 62-year-old bank vice president, was worried about her memory. She couldn't recall the details of her accounts as well as she used to, and she'd even begun to miss appointments. During her first visit with me, she was uncomfortable turning off her phone—she had a pressing work issue and had to stay in touch with the office. She took three or four calls during our meeting, and there must have been a pinging sound every few minutes, signaling a new text message or e-mail. She kept apologizing, but was unwilling, or maybe just unable, to disconnect from her devices. In addition to her phone, she had her iPad and laptop computer next to her in her briefcase—just in case.

Valerie's high anxiety stemmed in part from her technology addiction as well as her chronic multitasking. When I asked her about the possibility that her constant online life was contributing to her stress, she got defensive and said that she used the technology to make her life more efficient so she could free up more time to enjoy herself after work. But in truth she wasn't enjoying herself. She was under extreme stress from her nonstop work, which she took home with her at night, and couldn't stop using her gadgets.

I learned that many of her worries about her memory began when she upgraded her cell phone, which was just too much for her to handle. Her life was so frenetic that she didn't really have time to learn how to use the new phone correctly, and this created even more stress for her. Since I

**Q:** People are always talking about cell phones causing brain tumors— what about Alzheimer's? Is there any connection?

**A:** Studies have shown conflicting results regarding a connection between cell phone use and risk for brain tumors. No research has shown that cell phone use increases the risk for Alzheimer's disease, but recent investigations suggest possible effects on brain activity. Dr. Nora Volkow and colleagues at the National Institute on Drug Abuse performed brain PET scans on 47 volunteers before and after cell phone exposure. They found that 50 minutes of exposure to cell phone radiofrequency signals caused significant increases in brain function in the area closest to the cell phone antenna.

happened to have the same phone, I told her that the store that sells them has weekend classes on how to use it. I also suggested that she try a gadget-free afternoon each weekend to give her brain a break. Another strategy was to take a ten-minute break at work when she became anxious from multitasking. She followed my advice, reduced her stress levels, and her memory improved.

Valerie's experience is shared by many baby boomers who notice age-related memory changes and feel overwhelmed by all the new technology in their lives. These devices are meant to make our lives more efficient and even augment our biological memories. However, as they lure us into multitasking, they give us the perception of greater mental efficiency, but that perception comes at a cost. Recent research indicates that multitasking may lead to faster work, but with more errors—we actually become less efficient, having to go back and repeat tasks that weren't done correctly the first time. Whenever I have a tight deadline on a writing assignment, I make a point of turning off all my devices except those necessary to complete the task. Without the distractions, I get a lot more done in a shorter period of time.

One of the problems of multitasking is that although it seems like we're getting more done, our brains require time to switch from one task to another—an inefficient process. Dr. David Meyer and associates at the University of Michigan found that when study subjects quickly switched mental tasks between identifying shapes and solving math problems, both tasks took longer and accuracy declined compared to when the volunteers simply focused their attention on one task at a time.

Many people get hooked on a form of multitasking known as continuous partial attention. Rather than just switching from task to task, they are constantly monitoring and partially attending to multiple devices, hoping for the next bit of exciting stimulus. So even if they are writing an important paper or letter, part of their brain is continually scanning their immediate technological environment, searching for the most compelling ping or buzz signaling an important text or e-mail.

The process puts their brain on high alert and can lead to mental fatigue and distraction. Under mental stress, the brain will signal the adrenal gland to secrete cortisol and adrenaline to further boost energy levels and augment memory, but when this mental state becomes chronic, it can actually impair memory capacity, altering the neural circuitry in the brain regions that control mood and thought.

## Meditation Can Rewire Your Brain

I've met many people who swear by the benefits of meditation. They often seem calm and serene, and even those who still experience stress report that meditation helps them cope with that stress.

Neuroscientists now have evidence that meditating helps reduce stress and improve mental focus. Dr. Britta Hölzel and associates at Harvard Medical School recently put volunteers on a mindfulness meditation program. The study subjects meditated 30 minutes a day, using a form of meditation involving focused attention on sensations that include deep breathing and learning to bring the mind back to the breathing if it wandered off. MRI scans taken at the beginning and after eight weeks of meditating showed that the subjects had increased the volume of gray matter in the hippocampus, a brain area that controls learning and memory. The nonmeditating control group showed no change in hippocampal size.

Meditation also fires up the frontal areas of the brain that are associated with attention and

Q: Whenever I try to meditate, I get too antsy and I give up. What else can I do to reduce my stress?

A: Meditation is not for everyone. Some people find that when they combine physical movements with mindfulness, it not only relaxes them but also relieves their stress. You could try massage therapy, yoga, tai chi, a casual walk, or even an exercise class as alternative ways to reduce stress.

relaxation, and in people with memory loss it improves performance on challenging memory tests. After just three months of meditation training, volunteers became better able to release thoughts that popped into their minds, improving their ability to focus attention. Meditation not only strengthens the brain's memory and attention centers, but it also appears to fortify the neuronal circuits that control our emotions. Brief meditation breaks throughout the day or week can result in a sense of calm that often improves a person's feeling of well-being.

## MEDITATION: GETTING STARTED

GET COMFORTABLE AND CLOSE YOUR EYES. Breathe deeply and slowly. Focus on your breath and let your entire body relax.

YOUR MIND MAY WANDER. When it does, remind yourself that this is normal and simply bring your attention back to your breathing.

FOCUS YOUR ATTENTION ON A WORD OR MANTRA. This is another way to help bring your mind back from wandering.

BUILD YOUR MEDITATION SKILLS GRADUALLY. Set your timer for three minutes at first, and keep increasing your time until you work up to 30-minute sessions.

# Other Ways to Manage Stress

There are several approaches to develop effective habits for stress management, and no one method fits all. Here are a few strategies you might consider trying.

RUN FOR YOUR LIFE. Aerobic exercise routines not only build and protect brain memory centers, but they also help manage stress. A runner's high lifts our mood thanks to the natural brain endorphins released during a jog or power walk. You can enjoy the same mood boost from any form of cardiovascular conditioning, including swimming, tennis, basketball, and soccer. Many people find that their daily stress levels diminish rapidly from a physical workout.

I often recommend taking a brisk walk in the evening after dinner with a friend or spouse. You'll not only increase blood flow to your heart and brain, but you'll have a chance to talk about your day and share your frustrations, which often helps diminish them.

Many middle-aged and older people are challenged by possible injuries from wear and tear on their joints. They're often able to manage these kinds of issues by varying their workouts. For sore knees, switching from a treadmill to the elliptical machine or stationary bicycle may help avoid aggravation of sore joints and still provide a healthy aerobic workout. Also, changing your workouts offers additional benefits by exercising your brain and body differently.

DON'T GO SOLO. Most of us have trouble asking for help—often we fear that people will let us down and we'll feel rejected. However, if we take a chance and ask, we can be surprised by the willingness of others to pitch in and pick up some of the load. And if they can't help, we're no worse off than before. Social isolation increases an individual's risk for depression, so it's important to stay connected with friends and family to reduce stress. A recent UCLA study found that anticipated rejection can increase inflammation in the body, triggering the immune system to anticipate an attack or injury. Finding and keeping good and supportive friends is vitally important to minimizing stress and protecting the brain.

**TRY THIS!**

**BEACH FANTASY.** Close your eyes and imagine yourself on a beautiful beach. Feel a cool breeze and the sun on your skin. Sink your toes into the sand. Envision all the details of the experience as you continue to breathe deeply and drift into a state of relaxation. Don't worry about burning your skin—after all, this is a fantasy.

TAKE REGULAR BREAKS. Thanks in part to our high-tech lifestyles, a lot of us are spending considerable time in front of our computers, which can stiffen joints, tighten muscles, overwork our brains, and stress us out. Make a point of taking regular work breaks—away from the computer. Try turning off all your devices, including your cell phone and work tablet. Use the time to do something physical, maybe take a walk or stretch, or else just kick back and have a conversation with a coworker or friend (you can use the phone if necessary). If you like to meditate, do it. Or just find a quiet place and relax.

**TRY THIS!**

ABDOMINAL BREATHING. Get comfortable and breathe slowly and deeply. Expand your rib cage as you inhale initially, but after that, feel your abdomen rise with each breath. Stay relaxed and calm and breathe slowly throughout the exercise.

YOGA AND TAI CHI. Some people have a hard time sitting still and meditating and prefer incorporating physical movements into their relaxation routines. Yoga is an excellent option that integrates sequences of poses and breathing exercises that not only help us relax but also improve balance and flexibility.

Tai chi reduces stress and increases strength and balance through its systematic movements that require focused attention. Some of the movement sequences resemble martial arts in slow motion. They are low impact and do not stress the joints, so injuries are unlikely.

Tai chi helps reduce fatigue and pain and has been found to improve sleep in research volunteers suffering from fibromyalgia. Researchers at the Chinese University in Hong Kong reported that study volunteers who practiced tai chi exercises experienced improved cognitive functioning compared to a control group that did only stretching and toning. Dr. Michael Irwin and colleagues at UCLA have demonstrated that tai chi can boost immune function in older adults, making them less susceptible to infections.

SET REALISTIC GOALS. Some people tend to make lofty plans, but they are not always realistic about how much they can truly achieve. Setting unattainable goals is a common source of self-inflicted stress. It is possible to change this habit, but it requires slowing down and planning more reasonable goals.

If setting unrealistic goals is an issue for you, begin by simply looking at what you plan to do tomorrow. Make a list of all your tasks. See if you can delete, delegate, or postpone one or two of the items. Take note of whether this lowers your stress level for that day.

THINK AHEAD. Much of the stress or anxiety we experience comes from feeling a lack of control in our lives. Often we feel this way because we have failed to plan ahead.

My father used to tell me to "prepare 110 percent." At first I couldn't figure out his math, but eventually I realized the wisdom of his advice. By studying 10 percent more than I thought I needed to, I felt much more confident when I took an exam, gave a speech, or did whatever task I was anticipating with anxiety. A little extra prep didn't take away all the stress I was experiencing, but it helped diminish it.

This kind of preparation can apply to many situations, not just tests or public speeches. For example, if you tend to get anxious in certain social situations, consider planning ahead by asking your friend or spouse for the names of people

Q: I heard that cell phones may protect my brain. Is that possible?

A: A study from the Florida Alzheimer's Disease Research Center, in Tampa, offers evidence that cell phone exposure might benefit the brain. Dr. Gary Arendush and colleagues exposed laboratory mice that were genetically engineered to develop Alzheimer's disease to electromagnetic waves generated by cell phones. Some of the mice already had dementia, while others did not, so the scientists could test the effects on prevention of the disease as well as on the disease once it had developed. They found that seven to nine months of exposure for two hours each day protected the mice from memory impairment and reversed symptoms in mice that already had the disease.

**FULL BODY RELAXATION.** Close your eyes and breathe deeply as you systematically focus your attention on relaxing every muscle in your body. Begin with your head and scalp, and imagine releasing all the tension there. As you continue to breathe deeply, move your attention to your facial muscles and let them relax. Continue to move down your entire body. Take your time and enjoy the pleasant sensation of your whole body relaxing. Once you finish at your toes, try to envision yourself floating to the ceiling. Be sure to stop before you hit the ceiling.

who might be there. Nearly 10 percent of the population suffers from some form of social anxiety, which can be a risk factor for depression.

LAUGH OUT LOUD. Everyone enjoys a good laugh. It puts our worries in perspective and helps us distance ourselves from our concerns. Sometimes seeing the humor in our own everyday struggles can provide us with insight that can reduce our stress.

In addition to these psychological benefits, humor has physiological effects on the brain. Functional MRI studies have shown that humor activates the brain regions that control memory function, and the extent of the amusement people experience correlates to the degree of brain activity.

USE YOUR WORDS. Despite the lingering stigma of psychotherapy and psychiatric treatment, talk therapies have been found to reduce stress and help people with a range of stress-related psychological conditions, ranging from obsessive-compulsive disorder to clinical depression. Various forms of therapy appear to help specific psychological struggles. For example, people with phobias or obsessions often respond well to cognitive-behavioral therapy, a goal-oriented form of treatment based on the idea that patients' feelings and behaviors are caused by their own thoughts rather than by external events, situations, and relationships. Other patients with depression and anxiety do well with psychodynamic therapy, which explores the underlying psychological causes of their stress and helps them gain insight into their motivations, feelings, and behaviors.

Not everybody needs a therapist to get help with their problems. You can talk about feelings with anyone you trust: a friend, spouse, sibling, parent, priest, rabbi, or imam. We often get a sense of relief from airing our worries, and when the person listening does not judge or criticize us, we are able to experience their empathic response, and that soothing empathy can reduce our stress, help heal our emotional pain, and keep our brains healthy.

"IF I KNEW I WAS GOING TO LIVE THIS LONG, I'D HAVE TAKEN BETTER CARE OF MYSELF."

—MICKEY MANTLE

## CHAPTER 8

# Latest on Health Care and Medicine

MY TEENAGE SON STILL TEASES ME about the vacation we took a couple of years ago when he brought his skateboard to the resort. After lunch one day, I mentioned that I used to be a great skateboarder when I was his age, and I took him up on his dare to show him how good I still could be. Two minutes later, we were all piled in the rented mini-van, looking for the closest urgent care facility to get my sprained ankle wrapped. It didn't feel right for months.

Although numerous advances in medical technology

have allowed us to live longer, with age our bodies don't heal as quickly and we're more likely to develop chronic medical conditions. We do, however, have lots of medicines to manage these conditions and control their symptoms. Unfortunately, taking multiple medicines may cause side effects from drug interactions. My office staff knows to anticipate this common problem called polypharmacy, and they ask new patients to bring all their medications and supplements to their first appointment so that we can discuss them.

Recently 56-year-old hotel executive Bob L. and his wife came to my office. He was carrying a large briefcase and appeared tired and a bit older than his age. Bob said, "I've been having trouble sleeping for a while now, especially when I travel for work, and it's starting to affect my memory."

His wife jumped in. "And he keeps repeating himself over and over again."

He looked at her, annoyed. "Everybody does that. You do it, too. It drives me crazy."

After collecting some background information, I learned that Bob didn't have any obvious risk factors for Alzheimer's disease, such as a family history; and at age 56 he was rather young to begin developing symptoms of dementia. Although there appeared to be stress in his marriage, I suspected something else was contributing to Bob's memory issues.

I asked him about the medicines he was taking. He set his briefcase on my desk and opened it up. It looked like a portable pharmacy inside, with pill bottles practically spilling out.

I half-jokingly said, "That's all?"

His wife reached into her purse and pulled out several containers of supplements. "He takes these, too."

I sorted through the array of bottles and learned that Bob was taking a cholesterol-lowering statin, an antihypertensive, the antidepressant Paxil, the anti-inflammatory drug Motrin, Valium, and Prilosec to help his stomach, as well as a huge assortment of vitamins and supplements including melatonin, vitamins E, D, and C, fish oil, and several herbs with Chinese labels that I couldn't read.

Bob was one of those people with the best of intentions, trying to use medicines and supplements to keep his brain and body healthy. But he was operating on his own, based on partial information gathered from the Internet, TV morning shows, and magazine articles. His prescriptions were from various doctors who didn't necessarily know about all his other medicines.

Bob did need his antihypertensive to control his blood pressure, but he didn't have high cholesterol or arthritis. He was taking the statin and Motrin only because he read somewhere that they might lower his risk for Alzheimer's. That was also why he was taking high doses of various vitamins and supplements.

It turned out that the Paxil Bob took for depression was keeping him up at night, and the Valium he was taking for his insomnia could be contributing to his forgetfulness. I got him to stop taking the Motrin, and as a result, he no longer needed the Prilosec for the upset stomach the Motrin was causing. I also switched him from Paxil to a less stimulating antidepressant, so he no longer needed the Valium for sleep. Within a few weeks, Bob noticed a big improvement in his memory.

## Your Doctor Is Your Partner: No Secrets

Fortunately for Bob, he did not have Alzheimer's disease or any type of dementia. Once we figured out what medicines he really needed and changed or stopped the ones that were causing side effects, his memory symptoms improved.

Bob faced a problem shared by many people—poor communication with his doctors. He was taking some medications he didn't really need, prescribed by several different doctors, but no one physician was in charge, looking at the big picture of Bob's medical care.

A recent survey from the Alzheimer's Foundation of America national memory screening program found that most people don't even discuss their memory issues with their doctors. Of the more than 2,100 volunteers surveyed, nearly 70 percent experienced memory complaints, but only 21 percent of them had discussed those complaints with their doctors. Nearly half the respondents had seen their doctor within the previous six months, yet they still failed to communicate their memory issues with them.

Q: **I've become more forgetful over the last few years. My doctor says I don't have Alzheimer's, but I wonder if I should start taking an anti-Alzheimer's drug anyway. Could it help or possibly hurt me?**

A: Results of anti-Alzheimer's drug investigations in people without dementia have been mixed. Because the more severe forms of mild cognitive impairment put people at a higher risk for Alzheimer's dementia, some doctors have been treating their patients with these drugs. Some, but not all, people with mild cognitive impairment who take these medicines experience a benefit. It is sometimes difficult to tell if that benefit is a real effect or a placebo effect.

Thanks to the Internet and other media, many people are becoming savvier health care consumers. They gather the latest information on medical research, medications, herbal supplements, and what appear to be treatment breakthroughs, often before their own doctors have had time to study them. However, this constant influx of medical data can often be conflicting and difficult to sort through without the help of an informed physician.

The Pew Internet & American Life Project reported that 80 percent of U.S. Internet users have searched for health information online, and this information influences whether or not they turn to their doctor for help. Unfortunately, many people fail to check the reliability of what they've read, so they are often misinformed about their health care. Your doctor can help you make sense of the data and determine what is real and what may be hype or distortion.

The goal is to partner with your doctor and develop a relationship where you can ask questions, get answers, and share the decision making about what is best for your health. When doctors proactively involve patients in clinical decisions by openly discussing potential risks and benefits of treatment options, patient satisfaction increases significantly.

Lisa K., a 63-year-old travel agent, told her friend about how much she adored her family doctor. She went on and on about what a genius he was, how he graduated first in his class at Harvard Medical School, and now that he was divorced, he'd be perfect for her daughter.

When her friend asked about Lisa's health, Lisa mentioned the cardiologist she was seeing about her heart arrhythmia, the chiropractor and acupuncturist who were treating her back pain, the gastroenterologist who had diagnosed her gastric reflux disorder, and the neurologist who had just prescribed a new medicine to help with her memory problems. Her friend asked how her family doctor managed to coordinate all these specialists. Lisa said that she would never tell him about all these other doctors and hurt his feelings like that.

Lisa's problem was not unlike Bob L.'s. She was seeing too many doctors and taking multiple medications, without guidance on how her medicines interacted and might be causing side effects. She needed to come clean to her primary physician, who could then manage all her conditions, specialists, and medications.

Many patients like Lisa are reluctant to talk openly with their doctors. They may hide the fact that they went to get a second opinion, believing it might insult their doctor. Or perhaps they haven't been taking their medication as prescribed and feel they will disappoint their doctor, who might disapprove of their poor compliance.

If you want the best medical care, it's important to be candid with your physician about everything, including any consultations you get and all the medicines that you take, including supplements. It's also important to have one primary-care doctor who serves as your main advocate—someone who manages all your conditions, consultations, and medications, and who makes sure that everyone involved is informed of all these things.

## Treating Physical Illness Protects Your Brain

Following your doctor's medical recommendations is an important healthy brain strategy to lower your risk for cognitive decline and dementia. Left untreated, heart disease, diabetes, and hypertension cause damage or injury to the brain's supporting blood vessels, the cerebrovascular system. Hypertension and diabetes sometimes lead to tiny strokes in the hippocampus, one of the first memory centers affected by Alzheimer's disease, and small strokes may contribute to cognitive losses.

These kinds of vascular changes can undermine brain health. Our UCLA research group used functional MRI scanning to determine whether risk factors for vascular disease affected brain function in middle-aged and older volunteers. We found that higher blood pressure correlated with greater brain activation during memory tasks. This increase in brain activity may be how the brain compensates for subtle injuries to memory centers due to even slight increases in blood pressure.

Treatment of hypertension can protect your brain. A study of more than 1,300 older hypertensive volunteers found that those using antihypertensive medication for four years had significantly

## TIPS FOR GETTING THE MOST OUT OF YOUR DOCTOR VISIT

PREPARE YOUR QUESTIONS IN ADVANCE. Many patients get anxious during their doctor visit and forget to mention important concerns. Before your appointment, make a list of your most pressing issues and include notes about specific memory changes you might be experiencing.

TAKE IN NEWSPAPER OR INTERNET ARTICLES. Your doctor can help you put the headlines into perspective so you can understand how they apply to you.

TAKE ALONG ALL YOUR MEDICINES. If several doctors are prescribing for you, take in all your medicines, or at least a list of them, to review with your doctor. Don't forget the medicines you're not using anymore, as well as any over-the-counter drugs and supplements you may be taking.

SHOW UP EARLY FOR YOUR APPOINTMENT. You may need to fill out forms before meeting with the doctor; if you get there early, you and your physician won't be rushed during the visit.

DISCUSS NONMEDICAL ISSUES. Lifestyle choices are crucial to your brain health. Discuss your diet, exercise, stress management, and brain fitness habits.

MAKE YOUR NEXT APPOINTMENT. Before leaving the office, don't forget to make your next appointment, even if it's just for your next check-up.

less vascular brain disease than those who did not take their medicines. People with mild cognitive impairment who receive treatment for diabetes, high blood pressure, and high cholesterol are 40 percent less likely to develop Alzheimer's disease compared with those who have these conditions and don't receive treatment.

Nearly two thirds of people 70 and older have hearing loss, which also appears to increase the risk for developing Alzheimer's disease. Researchers at Johns Hopkins in Baltimore found that for people age 60 or older, hearing loss accounted for 36 percent of their risk for dementia. The social isolation resulting from hearing loss may explain this increased dementia risk, but many forms of hearing loss improve with implants or hearing aids, which could protect the brains of many older adults.

A wide range of physical conditions can also contribute to memory loss and mental symptoms. It can be as minor as a flu or urinary tract infection or possibly a metabolic problem such as thyroid imbalance or even anemia. Treating the underlying medical condition sometimes improves the cognitive symptoms, which can range from subtle to severe, possibly mimicking Alzheimer's disease but instead representing a reversible dementia.

## Can Medical Drugs Also Battle Alzheimer's?

Taking the right medicine to treat medical illnesses like hypertension, diabetes, and high cholesterol is critical to maintaining brain health. Some people, however, are taking these kinds of drugs even when they don't have high cholesterol or hypertension.

Bob L., the hotel executive who was worried about his memory, was taking a statin drug even though his cholesterol level was normal before he started to take the medicine. Dr. Christine Reitz and coworkers at Columbia University in New York found that when people have very high blood levels of HDL, the so-called good cholesterol, their risk for Alzheimer's was lowered by 60 percent compared to those with the lowest HDL levels. Although the use of statin drugs in

Q: **I'm confused by what I've heard in the news about estrogen replacement therapy. Can it prevent Alzheimer's disease in women?**

A: Large epidemiological studies have shown that women who used estrogen replacement therapy had a lower risk for developing Alzheimer's disease. This observation led to more studies. The largest was part of the Women's Health Initiative, and the researchers found that women age 65 or older who took Premarin (a brand of estrogen) actually had an increased risk of developing dementia. However, more recent research indicated that women taking hormone therapy only around the time of menopause (on average, age 49) had a 26 percent *lower* risk for dementia compared to a 48 percent *greater* risk for those taking hormones late in life (on average age 76). So the timing of estrogen replacement is what seems to make the difference in its potential to prevent dementia.

people with high levels of LDL (so-called bad cholesterol) does appear to lower their risk for developing Alzheimer's disease, it is not clear that this drug benefits people whose cholesterol levels are normal at the outset.

New research has found that the insulin used to treat diabetes may protect the brain from toxic amyloid proteins that damage brain cell connections. Another drug used to treat type 2 diabetes, rosiglitazone (Avandia), increases sensitivity to insulin and enhances its brain protective effect. These findings suggest that new drugs designed to increase insulin sensitivity could be a key to more effective anti-Alzheimer's treatments.

Because of initial evidence pointing to brain protective effects of anti-inflammatory drugs, some people take them for no other reason than to protect their brain health. However, these medicines have side effects. They can cause stomach bleeding and kidney problems. A recent study of more than 13,000 volunteers found that anti-inflammatory drugs, including ibuprofen (Motrin), naproxen (Aleve), and celecoxib (Celebrex), as well as aspirin, all lowered the risk for Alzheimer's disease. But this kind of association between using a medicine and having a lower future risk for Alzheimer's doesn't prove that the medicine is offering a true benefit. Only a placebo-controlled study can do that. Such studies of anti-inflammatory drugs have yielded mixed results in protecting brain health, so many doctors are reluctant to prescribe them unless there is a medical indication, such as arthritis or pain.

I routinely advise my patients to start exercising and eating a brain healthy diet. I know these strategies are safe and offer immediate health benefits, but like many doctors, I am more conservative about recommending medications that *may* lower an individual's risk for Alzheimer's disease but have side effects. I prefer waiting for more definitive studies so that patients don't put themselves at risk.

## Beware: Some Drugs Can Cause Dementia

Bob L. was taking Valium to help him sleep at night. Valium (diazepam) is in a group of anxiety-lowering medicines known as benzodiazepines. Although they are effective in calming people during the day and helping them sleep at night, they can impair memory in middle-aged and older people. For patients who can't get without this kind of medicine, switching from a long-acting benzodiazepine like Valium to a shorter-acting antianxiety medicine like Xanax (alprazolam) or Ativan (lorazepam) can help. Short-acting medicines are excreted from the body quickly and are less likely to accumulate in the brain and thereby cause memory side effects.

**TRY THIS!**

Shake up your brain cells by turning this book upside down and reading a sentence out loud.

Be sure to ask your doctor or pharmacist about over-the-counter drugs like Benadryl or Sominex before you start using them—you could head off a drug-induced dementia. These kinds of medicines for allergies and insomnia can cause memory side effects. They have an anticholinergic (diphenhydramine) that counteracts the cholinergic neurotransmitters, or brain messengers, that are important for learning and recall.

Drugs for illnesses like hypothyroidism can potentially impair memory and cause confusion and irritability. Medicines like prednisone or corticosteroids can have mental effects as well. By reviewing the timing of your medicine use and onset of memory complaints with your doctor, you can usually figure out which drug might be causing your memory symptoms.

Polypharmacy may lead not only to drug side effects but also to interactions between the drugs in your body, causing further problems. Your doctor's job is to work with you to limit unnecessary polypharmacy by stopping medicines that aren't necessary, avoiding the use of drugs to treat side effects of other drugs, and introducing nonpharmacological approaches whenever possible.

## Update on Supplements and Vitamins

Q: I know smoking can give a person lung cancer, but is it bad for your brain, too? Can it increase your risk for Alzheimer's?

A: Investigators at the University of California, San Francisco, recently reported on an analysis of multiple studies examining the relationship between smoking and Alzheimer's disease risk. They concluded that smoking is a significant risk factor for Alzheimer's. Other studies indicate that smoking increases the risk for vascular dementia caused by narrowing of the blood vessels in the brain. Many patients who develop dementia have a combination of Alzheimer's and vascular dementia, so kicking the smoking habit is definitely good for your brain.

I was at a health food store in my neighborhood recently, looking to buy some fish oil capsules and multivitamins. As I reached for a bottle to read the label, a woman started lecturing me on the benefits of water-soluble versus fat-soluble vitamins. I tried to tell her I knew that, but she wouldn't let me get a word in. She went into a discourse on how fat-soluble vitamins are stored in the body's fat cells and can build up over time and become toxic; whereas water-soluble ones are used by the body and then excreted by the kidneys right away. I told her I understood and thanked her for the information as I quickly headed for the produce. She yelled after me, demanding to read the labels on the vitamins I picked. Thanks to what Gigi calls my selective listening, I didn't appear to hear her.

An estimated 50 percent or more of adults take vitamins and supplements, yet many have only a vague idea of how these pills and capsules affect their brain health. One reason for the confusion is that vitamins and herbal remedies don't require the same level of scientific evidence for approval as that needed for a prescription drug. Therefore, consumers may be misled by promises made on the product containers. Also, people often assume that because they are ingesting something natural, it is safe, but that is not always true. Ginkgo biloba, a popular herbal supplement for memory loss, has been known to cause bruising or internal bleeding in people who also take blood thinners.

Despite such concerns, recent studies suggest promise for several dietary supplements that may protect brain health as we age. The challenge for consumers is to find reliable products, as well as sound information on both the potential benefits and drawbacks of a product.

## Curry in a Pill

Not everyone loves chicken curry or Indian food, so if you want to get the anti-inflammatory, antiamyloid, and antioxidant benefits of curcumin, the active ingredient in turmeric or curry, you might consider taking it in supplement form. It is not clear whether curcumin actually penetrates the blood–brain barrier and gets into the brain when taken in a pill form, so mixing it with omega-3 fats in cooking oils might optimize brain penetration.

Research from Nizam's Institute of Medical Sciences, in India, however, suggests that direct brain absorption may not be necessary for dietary curcumin to exert its brain protective effects. The investigators measured blood markers of inflammation of volunteers taking 150-milligram curcumin capsules twice a day. After eight weeks of treatment, they found significant reductions in several measures of inflammation in the body, and the cells that line blood vessels showed improved function. Maintaining normal blood vessel function is important for protecting the body from diabetes and strokes—conditions that can deteriorate brain health.

Even though curcumin may not be penetrating the blood–brain barrier, it may be exerting its effect by triggering the cells in the stomach lining to launch a general anti-inflammatory response throughout the body. The bottom line is that if you don't care for curried cuisine, or don't want to bother mixing your turmeric in with cooking oils, a capsule may be all you need to gain some brain protective benefits. Our

UCLA research team is conducting a double-blind placebo-controlled study to determine whether curcumin in a pill can also delay memory decline and the buildup of plaques and tangles in the brain.

## Phosphatidylserine

Phosphatidylserine is a nutrient we get from several foods, including tuna, herring, eel, and soy products. It serves as an important structural component of cell membranes throughout the body. Controlled studies using phosphatidylserine supplements have demonstrated its cognitive benefits in people with mild age-related memory complaints, as well as people suffering from dementia.

A recent double-blind study from Sourasky Medical Center, in Tel Aviv, Israel, used a combination of phosphatidylserine (300 milligrams daily) with the omega-3 fatty acid DHA in older adults with age-related memory complaints. After four months of treatment, the investigators found significant improvements in verbal memory abilities in the supplement group compared with a placebo group.

In another study, Japanese investigators used soybean-derived phosphatidylserine (but without DHA), also at 300 milligrams daily, and found that after six months of treatment, people with mild cognitive impairment (aged 50 to 69 years) had better memory performance compared to a group taking a placebo. Laboratory studies of phosphatidylserine suggest that it may protect brain health and improve cognitive performance by stabilizing brain cell membranes and improving the function of several brain neural transmitters that influence memory ability.

## Vitamin B Update

Although vitamin $B_{12}$ is abundant in fish, chicken, eggs, and many meats, not all adults absorb adequate amounts from their diet, so B vitamins are usually included in multivitamin supplements. Folate, or folic acid (an antioxidant B vitamin), is recommended during pregnancy to prevent fetal neural defects. It may also protect older adults from developing strokes and heart disease.

These two B vitamins as well as vitamin B$_6$ are involved in the breakdown of homocysteine, one of the amino acid building blocks of protein in the body. Scientists recently found that high levels of homocysteine in the blood increase the risk for Alzheimer's disease. Moreover, lower blood levels of these B vitamins and higher blood levels of homocysteine are associated with cognitive decline.

Oxford University investigators gave either daily B vitamins (folic acid, vitamin B$_{12}$, and vitamin B$_6$) or a placebo to study volunteers with mild cognitive impairment. After two years, those receiving the B vitamins had significantly less cognitive decline, and their MRI scans showed less brain shrinkage than the others' scans. The greatest response to the B vitamins was seen in volunteers with the highest homocysteine levels at the beginning of the study.

B vitamins are critical to the synthesis of DNA and protect brain health by maintaining neural cell integrity. A recent study found that vitamin B$_{12}$ may help the body control inflammation. Although some people take very high doses of B vitamins, megadoses of these vitamins have not been found to provide additional benefits compared to those conferred by normal doses, and taking megadoses poses the risk of side effects, including numbness in the hands and feet.

## The Upside of the Sun: Vitamin D

Even though sunlight and milk products provide healthy doses of vitamin D, many people are deficient in this vitamin because they spend much of their time indoors and use sunblock outdoors. Vitamin D not only keeps our bones strong and prevents fractures, it also protects brain health. Low levels of vitamin D are associated with extensive cognitive decline. In a study of more than 5,000 older women, those taking the recommended weekly amount of at least 35 micrograms of a vitamin D supplement had better cognitive ability than those who did not.

Q: I know someone who smoked a lot of marijuana during the 1960s and may still even continue this habit. Now he's turning 60 and complaining about his memory. Do you think that pot smoking caused damage to his brain?

A: Studies of moderate marijuana use do not show obvious cognitive effects. Tetrahydrocannabinol (THC) is the main ingredient of marijuana that causes the high that some people enjoy. A second chemical, cannabidiol, produces a calming effect. Subjects at the University of London who smoked cannabis low in cannabidiol showed difficulty on recall tests performed when not intoxicated; subjects who smoked cannabis high in cannabidiol showed no memory impairment on the test. People with prescriptions for medical marijuana might consider requesting strains high in cannabidiol in order to avoid memory effects.

## Antioxidant Vitamins

The Alzheimer's prevention program includes generous helpings of antioxidant fruits and vegetables. Many health enthusiasts recommend fighting off the brain-aging effects of oxidation by getting these vitamins through dietary supplements, but some have gone overboard with their beliefs in the health benefits of antioxidant vitamins. The brilliant chemist Linus Pauling, who won the Nobel Prize in Chemistry, was criticized for his scientifically unsubstantiated claims of the benefits of megadoses of the antioxidant vitamin C for protection against the common cold and cancer.

In the late 1990s Dr. Mary Sano and her collaborators reported that Alzheimer's patients who took 2,000 units of the antioxidant vitamin E had slower declines in everyday function compared with those taking placebo. Following that report, Alzheimer's experts started recommending high doses of vitamin E supplements for their patients. However, in 2005 Dr. Edgar Miller and colleagues reported that patients taking megadoses of vitamin E may increase their risk for heart attacks and even death. Today, few doctors advocate the use of over 400 daily units of vitamin E as a brain protection strategy.

Many antioxidant supplements, including acetyl-l-carnitine and coenzyme Q10, have demonstrated positive effects in laboratory and animal studies, but research confirming their ability to help prevent Alzheimer's disease in people has yet to be published. Studies of antioxidant supplements, including vitamins C and E, beta carotene, and flavonoids, have not shown consistent brain protective results. Our initial UCLA work with pomegranate juice, which contains polyphenol antioxidants, has shown cognitive improvements in people with mild memory changes, and studies of the brain and memory effects of pomegranate-polyphenol capsules are ongoing.

### Other Supplements That May Protect the Brain

Ginkgo biloba's antioxidant and brain circulation properties could explain the cognitive benefits observed in some studies of it in people with normal aging and in others with dementia. However, a recent large-scale study has raised questions about whether or not ginkgo biloba truly improves memory and brain health.

Docosahexaenoic acid (DHA), a form of omega-3 fatty acid, comes from many foods, especially fatty fish such as salmon, tuna, and mackerel. The cognitive and brain health benefits of DHA have been reported in people before they get dementia, whereas studies using DHA supplements in people who already have symptoms of Alzheimer's disease demonstrate no advantages beyond placebo treatment.

Our knowledge of supplements and herbal treatments for Alzheimer's prevention is still limited, so I like to keep an open mind about the possible benefits of some of the proposed interventions. A recent controlled study using a form of American ginseng demonstrated improvements in both cognition and mood in young adult volunteers. These kinds of preliminary reports are worth pursuing further, since not all forms of ginseng seem to show the same kinds of benefits.

# Anti-Alzheimer's Drugs

In the late 1980s, when I began studying Alzheimer's and caring for patients and families affected by the disease, doctors didn't have too much to offer patients. They emphasized careful diagnosis to identify pseudodementia depressions that might mimic Alzheimer's disease. In those situations, the anti-Alzheimer's drug was an antidepressant, which often improved mood and cognitive symptoms. We also searched for thyroid problems, and sometimes the anti-Alzheimer's drug was a synthetic thyroid medicine.

Q: **I have been taking a statin drug to lower my cholesterol for several years. I know that it may be lowering my risk for Alzheimer's disease, but my doctor says it may not help. How is that possible?**

A: Several large-scale studies, including a recent one involving more than 3,000 people age 75 years and older, indicate that statins slow the rate of cognitive decline and delay the onset of Alzheimer's disease in people with normal aging. However, for people who have Alzheimer's disease or dementia, statins have no apparent benefit.

It wasn't until the late 1990s that more specific treatments for Alzheimer's disease symptoms first became available. Because an Alzheimer's brain is deficient in acetylcholine (a memory neurotransmitter), drugs were developed to increase levels of acetylcholine. The first FDA-cleared cholinergic drug was tacrine (Cognex), but its side effects made it difficult to use. In 1996 an effective and more tolerable compound became available, and we now have three drugs that enhance acetylcholine in the brain: donepezil (Aricept), rivastigmine (Exelon), and galantamine (Razadyne). These medicines have been approved for use in patients with Alzheimer's disease, and they also help patients with other dementias (for example, vascular, Lewy body, and Parkinson's).

These drugs not only improve memory and thinking, but they can also reduce agitation, depression, and the burden of care for family members. Though side effects are usually minimal, some people experience loss of appetite, indigestion, nausea, slowed heart rate, or insomnia. Most doctors increase the medication dosage gradually in order to minimize side effects. Patients who get an upset stomach can use a patch form of rivastigmine that delivers the medicine through the skin. Once patients are stable on a cholinergic drug, doctors often add memantine (Namenda), a medicine that works on a different brain receptor and further boosts cognitive benefits.

# Is It Wise to Take Smart Drugs?

G igi and I visited Grandma Ollie shortly before she died at age 104. This was the first year ever that she hadn't sent Gigi a birthday card. I didn't suspect that Grandma had dementia, but perhaps she was getting mild cognitive impairment and could benefit from an antidementia medicine, a so-called "smart drug."

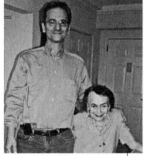

When we visited, she still looked physically healthy, but as you can see in the photo to the right, she continued to be height challenged.

To find out how she was doing mentally, I planned to casually slip in a few questions during the conversation. I began by asking her how old she was and she said, "Shut up, Gary." I knew right then, it was the same old Grandma Ollie I'd always known.

Whether people are beginning to have memory symptoms or not, they often want to know if it would be helpful to take anti-Alzheimer's drugs as smart drugs to help them with their middle-age pauses or senior moments. The evidence for using these medicines off-label—in other words, in a different way than that approved by the FDA—for mild memory complaints is mixed. One study of mild cognitive impairment found that patients taking donepezil (Aricept) were less likely to get Alzheimer's disease after a year of treatment compared to those taking placebo, but no drug advantage was found after three years. Despite such mixed results in controlled clinical trials, many doctors are using these medicines off-label—up to 44 percent of patients with mild cognitive impairment receive them.

For people with even milder forms of memory decline, some limited studies suggest possible benefits. Our UCLA group found that middle-aged and older adults with only mild memory complaints who took donepezil for 18 months had increased activity in some brain memory centers as seen on PET scans. Although their brain scans looked healthier, the volunteers who took donepezil did not have any cognitive benefits, including memory, compared to those taking placebo. Dr. Steven Ferris and colleagues at New York University found that in people with age-associated memory impairment, three months of treatment with memantine improved attention and the rate at which they could process new information compared with volunteers taking a placebo. The bottom line is that we don't yet have consistent evidence for using these medicines as smart drugs, but some individuals who take them experience temporary cognitive benefits.

## In Search of an Alzheimer's Cure

Available drugs for Alzheimer's can help with symptoms, but they don't cure the underlying disease. Although patients often experience temporary improvement, after a year or more the symptoms of the disease will still get worse. The temporary gains can be meaningful, however, often keeping patients at home with their families and delaying nursing home placement. Eventually, though, they reach a plateau in their medication response and gradually begin to decline at a rate that parallels the rate of decline that would have occurred had they never taken any medicine at all. In addition, if a symptomatic drug is stopped when the patient begins to gradually decline, the prior gains from the treatment are rapidly lost.

The Holy Grail for Alzheimer's drug development is to find a so-called disease-modifying medicine that slows the rate of cognitive decline and provides a sustained effect. Universities, research institutes, and pharmaceutical companies are investing considerable time and resources in searching for this kind of drug.

But it is no simple pursuit. It may take years of laboratory studies, followed by years of tests in patients, to discover and develop a safe and effective medication. This is one of the major reasons it is so important to do all that we can now to prevent the disease from attacking our brains.

In recent years, the pharmaceutical industry has focused considerable resources on developing drugs that target beta-amyloid plaques, one of the abnormal proteins that accumulate in the brains of Alzheimer's victims. These antiamyloid drugs have looked promising in animal studies and early clinical trials, but many have failed because of toxicity or lack of effectiveness in more advanced clinical trial testing. Some experts believe that testing these drugs once patients already have symptoms of dementia is too late in the disease process. It's possible that focusing studies on patients with mild cognitive impairment would be a more successful approach. Another strategy is to attack the building blocks of amyloid or its precursors, rather than the end result of amyloid plaque deposits.

Alzheimer's disease is not just an abnormality of amyloid deposits; many other normal structures and functions are breaking down in an Alzheimer's brain. Some scientists are targeting tau tangles. Dr. Ralph Nixon and colleagues at the Nathan Kline Institute, in New York, have shown that a major problem in the Alzheimer's brain is a defect in the way biological waste material is removed. His studies suggest that defective lysosome cells, the garbage collectors in the brain, should be targeted for drug development. His group was able to prevent cognitive decline in animals by improving the ability of lysosomes to degrade and process waste proteins.

Another drug development approach focuses on high-risk groups, like those with a proven genetic risk for Alzheimer's disease. People who inherit two copies of the APOE-4 gene have up to a tenfold greater risk of developing Alzheimer's disease than those without this genetic risk. Patients with Down syndrome are also being studied because practically all of them develop Alzheimer's disease by the time they reach middle age. Our UCLA research group recently found a highly significant correlation between the age of Down syndrome subjects and

Q: I just read about some kind of new nasal spray that's supposed to protect you from getting Alzheimer's disease. Is this a bunch of hype or is there any real science behind it?

A: Scientists at Tel Aviv University are in the process of developing a vaccine nasal spray to help protect people from developing Alzheimer's disease. In the animal studies conducted so far, the vaccine appears to repair blood vessels in the brain by activating the body's immune system. In addition to possibly staving off Alzheimer's disease, this nasal spray may help with symptoms once a patient gets the disease. Although the animal studies are promising, human trials have not begun, and it could take years to see if it really works.

the accumulation of plaques and tangles in their brains as measured by PET scanning.

I am optimistic that within the next decade, we will have more effective drugs for Alzheimer's disease prevention. Clinical trials are available throughout the U.S. and abroad (see www.clinicaltrials.gov for listings), and many of these studies now focus on mild cognitive impairment and normal aging to discover drugs that would delay the onset of Alzheimer's disease and ultimately prevent it. People who have a higher risk for dementia because of their family history may be particularly interested in getting involved as volunteers for a study in their area.

## Antidepressants for Memory and Mood

Symptoms of cognitive loss and depression often become intertwined. Sometimes people who are aware of their memory loss become frustrated and depressed about their declining cognitive capacities, but in other situations symptoms of depression may result from an underlying brain problem. Investigators from UCLA's Alzheimer's Disease Research Center recently found that depression in patients with mild cognitive impairment predicted a swift progression to Alzheimer's disease. Treatment with the anti-Alzheimer's drug donepezil delayed this progression to Alzheimer's disease in depressed patients but not in those without symptoms of depression.

Older depressed patients often display symptoms of cognitive decline. In fact, impaired concentration is one of the clinical features of a major depression regardless of someone's age. Responses to antidepressant drugs also vary: Some people improve in mood only, while others have greater benefits in cognition and clarity of thinking. Investigators at the Rotman Research Institute, in Toronto, Canada, used PET scanning to understand some of these differences and found varying neural circuitry activity according to the volunteers' responses to an antidepressant drug. Combined depression and confusion can have several underlying causes, and treatments need to be individualized to get the best results.

# Managing Your Health Care to Protect Your Brain

Medical matters become an increasing challenge as we age, but knowing about our health problems and what we can do about them can lower our risk for cognitive decline and Alzheimer's disease. Keep in mind the following strategies as you take control of your health care to protect your brain:

- Your doctor is your partner: Make sure that you cover all your health concerns and questions at every appointment. Keep no secrets, especially about your memory.

- If you have age-related illnesses, be sure to take your medicine as directed to reduce your risk for cognitive decline.

- Medication side effects can mimic dementia, so take all your medicines to your doctor appointment to systematically review your prescriptions and over-the-counter drugs.

- Vitamins and supplements offer promise as brain-protective strategies, but we still have more to learn more about them through ongoing research. Don't take larger doses than recommended, and don't substitute supplements for a healthy brain diet.

- Several anti-Alzheimer's drugs are available to treat dementia, but none has been proven effective for mild memory decline.

- Depression can mimic Alzheimer's symptoms. Getting accurate diagnoses and treatments may improve mood and memory.

**Q:** I recently read that a medicine used to prevent kidney transplant rejection stops Alzheimer's disease. Can I ask my doctor to write a prescription for me?

**A:** You are probably referring to rapamycin (Rapamune), a drug that suppresses immune function and is used to prevent rejection after organ transplantation. Studies of mice engineered to develop Alzheimer's disease indicate that rapamycin extends life span, improves memory ability, and reduces levels of toxic amyloid protein. These studies are encouraging but the drug still needs to be tested in human volunteers to determine whether these findings can be replicated. Rapamycin suppresses the immune system: Significant side effects include increased risk of developing cancer. It's always best to wait until the clinical research determines the true risks and benefits.

"THE MOST
IMPORTANT THING ABOUT
GETTING SOMEWHERE
IS STARTING
RIGHT WHERE WE ARE."

—BRUCE BARTON, AUTHOR,
ADVERTISING EXECUTIVE,
POLITICIAN

## CHAPTER 9

# Your First Seven Days

ALMOST EVERYONE I HAVE EVER MET has at some point expressed a desire to change something in their life—from becoming less impatient at work to kicking their junk food habit or perhaps getting back into shape. Some people have no difficulty achieving their goals—they come up with a plan, get right into it, and accomplish their aims. But not everyone can stop smoking on the first try or stick to a diet without an occasional slip.

Throughout my career I have not only been impressed by how our genetic makeup seems to drive our behavior, but also by how much a little bit of assistance and guidance can help people create new habits and let go of old, self-destructive ones. When we are trying to change something in our lives, it often takes strong motivation to get us started, but seeing positive results keeps us going. Positive results combined with practice can soon turn new behaviors into healthy habits.

According to a recent study published in the *European Journal of Social Psychology*, some people are able to form a new habit in just 18 days, while others require a few months or longer. For behaviors to become habits, it helps to perform them in consistent settings and at regular times so our brains are cued by the environment and require less conscious thought to initiate them. The hope is that soon the new healthy behaviors in the Alzheimer's prevention program will become automatic.

When people grasp the connection between how their lifestyle choices affect their health, they are more likely to embrace healthy habits for the long term. The research on forming habits also shows that initiating new healthy brain behaviors for the first time takes planning. This is why I have laid out in detail the first seven days of the Alzheimer's prevention program. People interested in protecting their brain from Alzheimer's disease often notice results quickly and experience a mental spark of motivation. That positive feedback fuels their motivation to continue with their new healthy behaviors so they soon become lifestyle habits.

Neuroscientists have been able to pinpoint brain regions that work together when this mental spark of behavioral change ignites. Not surprisingly, our primitive dopamine reward system and our thinking brain, the frontal lobe, work together to change our behavior.

In the first seven days of the Alzheimer's prevention program, you will be begin to notice changes; incorporating these strategies into your life over the years is what it takes to stave off Alzheimer's disease. Those first seven days of the program bring together the essential elements that will help you create new habits in your life. Our research group has found that people are more likely to continue their program beyond the first seven days if:

- *The exercises are fun.* Memory and brain games should provide a mental challenge that piques your interest and makes you want to play more; and the physical exercises should be invigorating.

The Alzheimer's prevention program includes enough variety and choices so that even people who don't like to exercise will find a way to incorporate the program's strategies into their daily routine.

- *The initial commitment is brief.* If I asked every reader to spend three hours a day doing brain teasers, I'd have very few takers. All I'm asking for is a few minutes a day for one week to get started.
- *People see results within a week.* And then the benefits *really* kick in.

**TRY THIS!**

Combined physical and mental training: Stand on one leg while counting backward from 100 by sevens. Then switch to the other leg and start counting backward again.

Before you know it, the Alzheimer's prevention program becomes habit-forming. For behavior to have an impact on brain health and on fending off disease, the longer you keep it up, the better. But to truly protect your brain health, the Alzheimer's prevention program must become a routine part of your life for years to come.

The following section of this chapter spells out the details of the first seven days of your Alzheimer's prevention program. It tells you when, what, and how to eat, exercise, stimulate your brain, and interweave stress reduction techniques, so that each of these elements can easily become part of your daily routine.

The program is designed to fit into most people's busy lives, but it can be easily adjusted to meet your specific needs. If you find that your schedule does not allow for a brain fitness or stress relief exercise in the afternoon, you could simply do it whenever you have more time.

The program's diet provides a nutritious balance of proteins, carbohydrates, and foods rich in antioxidants and omega-3 fats. If losing weight is one of your goals, then try to remain mindful of your own feelings of hunger and satisfaction—that is your body's natural feedback system to help you achieve your ideal body weight.

Where no specific serving portions are listed, use your good judgment. For instance, one or two tablespoons of salad dressing are usually plenty. Also, it's a good idea to drink a glass of water (6 to 8 ounces) with a snack or after physical exercise. And a nighttime snack should be tasty but not very filling.

The stretching and physical conditioning exercises are safe for most people and should be done at your own pace. Also, you may want to consider consulting your physician before embarking on this or any diet and exercise program.

To help you budget your time, I've included how long it takes to do each of the exercises. The extra-credit exercises are optional if you have additional time.

## Stocking Your Kitchen Before You Get Started

The following lists include the foods you'll need for the first week or more of your program. Amounts listed are per person. Substitutions for special dietary needs are easy—for example, nuts can be replaced by beans; or if you are allergic to seafood, chicken or vegetarian proteins are fine. If you prefer poached eggs instead of scrambled or hard-boiled, feel free to substitute.

Vegetarians should feel free to substitute about 6 ounces of basic lentil or bean stew for any of the meats. A half cup of red kidney beans mixed into a lunch salad will give you the protein you need. Other beans high in protein include black, pinto, and garbanzo beans and lentils. Veggie burgers whose first five ingredients are vegetables or whole grains (rather than bread or filler) are also fine. Quinoa is a terrific, protein-rich grain, and recipes abound online and in books. Avoid eating pasta more than once a week.

### FRESH PRODUCE

1 bunch spinach

2 red bell peppers

1 head broccoli

3 large carrots and 1 package baby carrots

1 bunch celery

1 head Romaine lettuce

1 head butter lettuce

1 bunch arugula

3 small red potatoes

1 Idaho potato

1 sweet onion

1 zucchini

1 pint cherry tomatoes

2 tomatoes

2 avocados

12 ounces blueberries

8 ounces strawberries

4 apples

1 bunch red and green seedless grapes

2 bananas

2 oranges

5 fruits (a combination of pears and peaches, if available)

1 grapefruit

2 lemons

15 ounces raisins

1 small can or jar each: artichoke hearts, olives, green beans

### DAIRY

1½ dozen eggs

six 4- to 6-ounce containers nonfat yogurt (at least 3 plain)

8 ounces string cheese, or sliced cheddar or Swiss if you prefer

8 ounces grated Parmesan cheese

1 pint low-fat cottage cheese

8 ounces low-fat cream cheese

1 quart nonfat milk

### MEAT/FISH

three 6-ounce boneless chicken breasts

two 4- to 6-ounce salmon fillets

4–6 ounces halibut

½ pound ground turkey

4–6 ounces sirloin steak

1 package turkey bacon

2–4 ounces sliced roast beef

2–4 ounces sliced turkey

2 ounces sliced smoked salmon

two 5- to 7-ounce cans tuna packed in water

### GRAINS/RICE/PASTA

assorted breads: whole wheat, rye, or sourdough; 1 bagel

1 package (6–8 breads) pita

1 small package corn tortillas

1 small box whole-grain crackers

oatmeal (regular or steel-cut)

8–12 ounces uncooked brown rice

## FROZEN

1 pint frozen yogurt

1 pint fruit sorbet

1 box frozen fruit-juice bars

## OTHER

six 6- or 8-ounce cans tomato juice or V-8

1 quart fruit juice (pomegranate if you like it)

36 ounces (2 cans) chicken soup with vegetables

11 ounces (1 can) tomato soup

8 ounces chopped walnuts

4 ounces unsalted almonds

1 pound popping corn (use an air-popper)

one 16-ounce jar chocolate sauce

1 small box teabags (green is optimal)

2 bottles sparkling water (or flat water)

1 small canister of decaf iced tea

1 bottle of wine if desired

## CONDIMENTS

1 small jar salsa

one 10-ounce jar all-fruit jam

1 small bottle extra virgin olive oil

1 small bottle balsamic vinegar

1 small bottle light vinaigrette dressing

1 small bottle light Caesar dressing

1 small bottle light ranch dressing

1 small jar light mayonnaise

*(If you'd like to make your own dressing or use just one type, that's fine)*

## FREEBIES (I.E., AS MUCH AS YOU LIKE)

green tea

sugarless gum

all herbs and spices, including fresh parsley, cilantro, dill, garlic, cinnamon

onions

sparkling or flat water

celery, cucumbers, bell peppers, spinach, broccoli

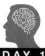

**WAKE-UP STRETCH AND CONDITIONING (2 minutes)**

First thing in the morning, do the following stretches and exercises:

STRETCH #1: SQUAT AND REACH STRETCH. Stand with your feet shoulder width apart. Raise your arms straight up above your head. Swing your arms forward and down behind you as you squat as low as possible. Then swing your arms forward and up above your head as you stand up and balance your body with your feet, hips, and shoulders aligned. Hold for 3 seconds. Repeat 4 times.

CONDITIONING EXERCISE # 1: RUSSIAN DANCER KNEE LIFTS. Stand upright and fold your arms in front at shoulder height like a Russian folk dancer. Lift your right knee toward your right elbow, and then alternate, bringing your left knee toward your left elbow. Exhale as the knee comes up, inhale as it goes down. Total: 10 per side.

**DRINK A GLASS OF WATER.**

**BREAKFAST**

*½ grapefruit*
*¾ cup hot oatmeal with 1 tablespoon raisins or walnuts (if you like)*
*½ cup nonfat milk or yogurt*
*Tea, coffee, or sparkling juice*
*(1 part fruit juice plus 2 parts sparkling water over ice)*
*Added refined sugar is not okay.*

**TIP FOR THE DAY**

We can't eliminate all the stress from our lives, but we can attempt to manage it better. Try anticipating any potential stress for today so you can take measures to avoid it. For example: leave a few minutes early for work so you don't have to worry about being late if you get stuck in traffic. You may not notice immediate benefits, but stress reduction has an impact on long-term brain health.

## MORNING MENTAL WARM-UP

Try doing the crossword puzzle, Sudoku, or KenKen puzzle in the newspaper. (Keep in mind, Monday is usually the easiest and the difficulty increases throughout the week.)

Notice some details of the clothing (color and pattern of a blouse, shirt, tie, etc.) of a family member, roommate, or the first person you see that day. Write those details on a piece of paper and put the note in your pocket or purse.

## AEROBICS ON THE GO (5 minutes)

Spend 5 minutes walking briskly outside or on a treadmill, cycling, or doing an aerobic workout of your choice before work or first errand of the day.

OR

Park or get dropped off a few minutes away from your first destination, and walk briskly the rest of the way.

## DRINK A GLASS OF WATER WHEN YOU ARRIVE.

## MIDMORNING SNACK

*1 cup nonfat plain or flavored yogurt with*
*2 tablespoons chopped walnuts mixed in*
*Green tea or water*

## MIDMORNING BRAIN TRAINING (4 minutes)

LOOK, SNAP, CONNECT. The three basic memory skills can be used to help remember people's names, appointments, shopping lists, or almost any everyday memory challenge:

1. <u>LOOK:</u> Focus your attention on what you want to recall later.

2. <u>SNAP:</u> Form a visual image or mental snapshot of the information you want to learn.

3. <u>CONNECT:</u> Create visual associations to link up your mental snapshots for later recall.

Use this technique to associate the following unrelated word pairs. First, *LOOK* by focusing your attention and studying the word pair for a moment or two. Then imagine a picture or *SNAP* for each word. Finally, *CONNECT* or link the images together. For example, I link together the word pair "football—hammock" by imagining a football resting in a hammock. The associations can be logical or illogical—sometimes the more unusual the connection, the easier it is to recall later.

See how you do with the following word pairs:

**telephone — rabbit**
**fork — candle**
**papaya — ballerina**

---

**LUNCH**

*Garden salad with 3–6 ounces grilled chicken, vinaigrette dressing*
*2 whole-grain crackers*
*Sliced pear*
*Iced tea or sparkling water with lemon*

---

**AFTERNOON STRESS RELIEF (3 minutes)**

Sit comfortably, close your eyes, and breathe slowly. Visualize your breath as it enters your sinuses, flows down into your chest, and expands your rib cage. Slowly exhale through your nose, following your breath as it rises through your chest and sinuses and finally leaves your body. Repeat slowly for 2 to 3 minutes.

## AFTERNOON SNACK

*1 ounce semifirm cheese of your choice*
*(e.g., string, cheddar, Swiss, Monterey Jack)*

## AFTERNOON BRAIN TRAINING (1 minute)

Write down the clothing details that you committed to memory before leaving the house this morning. Check the piece of paper in your pocket to see how you did. For extra credit, you might want to compliment that person on his or her fashion choice when you get home.

## DINNER

*Tossed green salad with balsamic vinegar and olive oil dressing*
*Grilled 6-ounce salmon filet with herbs and lemon slices*
*½ cup brown rice*
*Steamed spinach*
*Fruit sorbet*
*Decaf iced tea, sparkling water, and/or a glass of wine*

## EVENING AEROBICS/STRESS RELIEF (10 minutes)

Take a 10-minute after-dinner walk, followed by drinking a glass of water. If circumstances do not permit a walk, repeat this morning's Wake-Up Stretch and Conditioning routine.

**EVENING BRAIN TRAINING (2 minutes)**

When we create mental snapshots, elaborating visual detail helps us make them more memorable. Try this exercise to improve your skill:

Close your eyes and remember something you noticed during the day—it could be a car you saw, a room you were in, or a person you met. Spend a few moments recalling as many details of the memory as you can to enrich the mental image.

Now that you're warmed up, see how well you remembered the word pairs from this morning. Below are the first words; say the second word to yourself.

telephone _____

fork _____

papaya _____

**NIGHTTIME SNACK**

*Red or green seedless grapes*

### WAKE-UP STRETCH AND CONDITIONING (3 minutes)

STRETCH #1: SQUAT AND REACH STRETCH (see Day 1). Repeat 4 times.

STRETCH #2: SIDE STRETCH. Stand with feet shoulder width apart, knees slightly bent. Raise your right hand overhead and lean directly over your left side. Reach as far to the left as you can, then hold for a count of 5. Slowly bring your torso upright, then lower your arm. Raise your left arm overhead and lean to the right, reaching to the right side as far as you can. Hold for a count of 5. Slowly return to upright. Total: once per side.

CONDITIONING EXERCISE #1: RUSSIAN DANCER KNEE LIFTS (see Day 1). Total: 10 per side.

### DRINK A GLASS OF WATER.

### BREAKFAST

*Vegetable omelet (1 whole egg plus 2 egg whites
and fresh chopped vegetables)
½ cup of fresh blueberries (You can substitute frozen berries—
let them melt in your mouth like a candy or
toss them in a blender with ice for a small slushy.)
Tea or coffee (with milk and sweetener if you like) or sparkling juice*

### MORNING BRAIN TRAINING (5 minutes)

MEMORY HABITS. Memory habits remind us to take our vitamins at breakfast and brush our teeth after meals. To improve your everyday recall, learn the following memory habit to help you avoid having forgetful moments. Before leaving home, take a moment to think about what you have planned for the day. Review your daily calendar and make sure you haven't forgotten an appointment or something you might need later, such as a file, receipt, or package. To help make this a routine, try doing it at the same time and place each morning. I like to check the calendar in my cell phone when I first wake up—it also gives me a few more minutes in bed.

NAMES AND FACES. To further build your brain power, use *LOOK, SNAP, CONNECT* to learn the name of at least one person you meet today. Look carefully at the person's face and think about what their name sounds like or means. Also, take a mental snapshot of the face and connect the name-snap to the face-snap using a striking facial or body feature (e.g., Rosa has rosy cheeks or Jim looks like he works out at the gym). This can be someone you see every day when you're getting coffee or parking your car. Most people appreciate being asked their name, so don't be shy.

EXTRA CREDIT:
Do the crossword, Sudoku, KenKen, or puzzle of your choice.

**TIP FOR THE DAY**

Your posture affects both your physical and mental states; some studies have even shown that it can have a positive effect on memory. Good posture (belly and buttocks tight, head up, and shoulders back) not only changes your appearance and breathing, but it can also increase your confidence. Check your posture in the mirror before leaving home and try to remain mindful of your posture throughout the day, whether you're walking, standing, or sitting.

**AEROBICS ON THE GO (5 minutes)**

Spend 5 minutes walking briskly outside or on a treadmill, cycling, or doing an aerobic workout of your choice before starting your day.

OR

Park or get dropped off at least a few minutes away from your first destination and walk briskly the rest of the way.

Skip the elevator and take the stairs for at least a few flights. If there are no stairs, increase your pace as you walk toward your destination.

**DRINK A GLASS OF WATER WHEN YOU ARRIVE.**

---

**MIDMORNING SNACK**

*Hard-boiled egg (or whites of 3 hard-boiled eggs)*
*4 ounces baby carrots*
*Green tea or sparkling water*

---

**MIDMORNING BRAIN TRAINING (4 minutes)**

STORY METHOD. Let's use *LOOK, SNAP, CONNECT* with the *story method* to strengthen neural circuits for remembering unrelated words. Learn this technique and you will become a master of the shopping list—impress your friends and family. The following is an example of a list of unrelated words to remember:

pancakes
skateboard
grandmother
dishes
elf
football field

Here's the story I came up with: My *grandmother* made me *pancakes* before she *skateboard*ed past the *football field,* where she saw an *elf* juggling some *dishes.* There is no one correct story and you don't need to remember the words in order. Often your first association helps you remember the words better. Perhaps your story might have you washing the dishes after you ate your pancakes, or maybe your grandmother tossed the pancakes over to a juggling elf who served the breakfast to you on a football field.

Now try this method yourself. Memorize the following words by creating a story in your mind linking them together. Use your imagination and infuse the story with action and detail to make it more memorable. You might ask friends or family members to join in with their own list of words for you to remember.

teenager

oven

convertible

lawn

ticket

ocean

## LUNCH

*Tuna sandwich on whole wheat toast, with lettuce, tomato, light mayo*
*Crisp apple*
*Iced tea or sparkling water with lemon*

## AFTERNOON STRESS RELIEF (3 minutes)

Sit comfortably, close your eyes, and imagine yourself at a beautiful beach just before sundown. Breathe deeply as you envision the sun setting. Feel the misty ocean breeze. Hear the seagulls and the waves. Visualize the sun touching the horizon as it begins to slip below it, bit by bit—now half, three quarters, almost gone, and finally it completely disappears. Take one more deep breath and exhale slowly. Open your eyes and enjoy the relaxed feeling.

**AFTERNOON SNACK**

*1 cup nonfat yogurt (frozen is fine)*
*1 pear or peach*
*Iced tea or sparkling water with lemon*

**AFTERNOON BRAIN TRAINING (1 minute)**

STORY METHOD. Do you remember your story for the list of six words from this morning? To help jog your memory, I don't know the last time my teenager mowed the lawn, but I know what he'd rather do on a sunny day. . . .

**DINNER**

*Tomato, avocado, and sweet onion salad*
*with olive oil and vinegar dressing*
*Grilled 6-ounce chicken breast with herbs*
*3 boiled red potatoes*
*Steamed or pan-roasted broccoli*
*Sliced strawberries drizzled with 1 tablespoon chocolate sauce*
*Sparkling water and/or a glass of wine*

**EVENING AEROBICS/STRESS RELIEF (10 minutes)**

Take a 10-minute after-dinner walk, or repeat this morning's Wake-Up Stretch and Conditioning routine.

**DRINK A GLASS OF WATER.**

**EVENING BRAIN TRAINING (5 minutes)**

NAME RECALL. Try to recall the name and face of one person you met today. Some names are easy to remember because they immediately bring a mental image to mind. If I meet Frank Lincoln, I can see him driving a *Lincoln* Continental while munching on a *frankfurter*. Now try to visualize images that the following names might represent:

**Jim Katz**

**Angela Howe**

**Bill Lyons**

MEMORY PLACES. To avoid the "disappearing keys act," we can make a habit of creating memory places and putting often-used items in those places every day. Start by creating memory places for objects you are most likely to misplace. If it's your keys, install a key hook by the door or in the kitchen. For your cell phone, perhaps a convenient desk drawer would work or you could recharge it at night next to your purse or briefcase. Glasses could go on your nightstand. I have a colleague who parks in the same space every day at work so he won't forget where his car is. Not a bad idea . . .

**NIGHTTIME SNACK**

*Frozen fruit-juice bar*

**WAKE-UP STRETCH AND CONDITIONING (3 minutes)**

STRETCH #1: SQUAT AND REACH STRETCH (see Day 1). Repeat 5 times.

STRETCH #2: SIDE STRETCH (see Day 2). Total: 5 times per side.

CONDITIONING EXERCISE #2: MARCHING SOLDIER. Stand upright and march in place, lifting your knees waist high. With each knee raise, inhale and swing your opposite arm straight forward, as far and high as possible, then behind you as you exhale and lower your leg to switch knees—getting a good rotation in the shoulder. Continue marching for a count of 20.

EXTRA CREDIT:

CONDITIONING EXERCISE #1: RUSSIAN DANCER KNEE LIFTS. Total: 15 per side.

**DRINK A GLASS OF WATER.**

**TIP FOR THE DAY**

Drinking six glasses of water every day helps you feel full enough to make it to the next meal. Placing bottles of water in handy places, like your car, desk, bedside, purse, or briefcase, will remind you to drink water throughout the day. If water straight-up bores you, try sparkling mineral water. Some vitamin waters contain calories and sweeteners, so plain or sparkling water is preferable. Some people like to chew sugarless gum between meals. It's safe and can alleviate cravings.

**BREAKFAST**

*Scrambled eggs (2 egg whites plus one whole egg) with*
*2 strips turkey bacon*
*1 slice sourdough or rye toast with all-fruit jam*
*½ cup fresh or frozen blueberries*
*Tea, coffee, or sparkling juice*

**MORNING BRAIN TRAINING (3 minutes)**

MEMORY HABITS. At the same time and place as yesterday, check your calendar and plan ahead for the day. Look around so you don't forget something you may need.

NAME AND FACE RECALL. Do you remember this person's name? You met her back in Chapter 4.

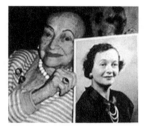

Try to learn two new names today. Remember that your associations don't have to be exact—use *LOOK, SNAP, CONNECT* as well as these tips:

- Repeat the name during your conversation. If the name is complex, long, or unusual, ask for the spelling and visualize it written out.

- As you visualize the name spelled out, focus on the face.

- Comment on how the person's name reminds you of someone else with that name.

- Ask about the person and concentrate on what you learn about their life while thinking about the name.

- Say the name when you say good-bye.

A bonus of this exercise is the extra social interaction it provides. Pushing yourself to meet new people challenges neural networks that control your social skills. Remember, a ten-minute conversation is probably a better brain booster than watching a *Law and Order* rerun.

EXTRA CREDIT:
Do the crossword, Sudoku, KenKen, or puzzle of your choice.

**AEROBICS ON THE GO (10 minutes)**

Spend 10 minutes walking briskly outside or on a treadmill, cycling, or doing an aerobic workout of your choice before starting your day.

OR

Park or get dropped off at least 10 minutes away from your first destination and walk briskly the rest of the way.

Skip the elevator and take a few flights of stairs. See if you can continue to increase the number of stairs you climb. If you have no stairs, increase your initial aerobic workout by a few minutes.

**DRINK A GLASS OF WATER WHEN YOU ARRIVE.**

**MIDMORNING SNACK**
*½ cup nonfat yogurt
with 1 tablespoon raisins mixed in
½ banana
Green tea or water*

---

**MIDMORNING BRAIN TRAINING (2 minutes)**

TIP-OF-THE-TONGUE. Try using the following exercise to conquer the annoying difficulty of recalling something that you're positive you know:

Keep a pad and pencil in your pocket or purse, or use the note function in your smart phone. The next time you have a tip-of-the-tongue moment, write down clues or phrases that remind you of the word, name, or title that you can't recall. If you remember it later, write it down in your pad or phone. If not, ask a friend or look it up in a book or on the Internet. Finally, use *LOOK, SNAP, CONNECT* to help you recall it next time.

See if you can come up with a list of four or more of these tip-of-the-tongue words over the next few days.

---

**LUNCH**

*Chicken soup with vegetables and 3–6 ounces white meat*
*½ pita bread, toasted*
*Orange sections*
*Iced tea or sparkling water with lemon*

---

**AFTERNOON STRESS RELIEF (2 minutes)**

FULL BODY RELAXER. Sit comfortably or lie down. Take a deep breath and let it out slowly. Close your eyes, and focus your attention on your head and scalp. Imagine releasing all the tension there. Move your focus down to your facial muscles, releasing any tension there. Let the relaxed feeling extend to your cheeks and jaw, down your neck and into your shoulders, releasing any tension there while continuing to breathe slowly. Continue relaxing through your arms, hands, abdomen, back, hips, legs, feet, and toes—releasing all tension. Keep breathing deeply for another minute, allowing every last bit of tension to leave your body as you exhale.

---

**AFTERNOON SNACK**

*½–1 cup raw vegetables, such as celery, red bell pepper, or carrots*
*plus 1 ounce light ranch dressing for dipping*
*1-ounce cheese of your choice (One slice of prepackaged*
*Swiss cheese is usually about an ounce.)*
*2 whole-grain crackers*

---

**AFTERNOON BRAIN TRAINING (1 minute)**

NAME AND FACE RECALL. Don't forget to learn some new names today. If you're still having trouble with it, here are some examples that might help.

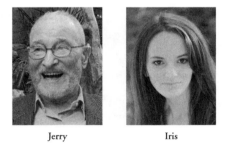

Jerry                    Iris

Jerry seems to be laughing it up and is quite merry—he seems like a *merry Jerry*. Iris has piercing brown eyes—her *irises* are quite remarkable. Your associations don't have to be exact. Often, just making the effort to focus on a distinguishing trait helps link the name to the face.

---

**DINNER**

*Butter lettuce salad with chopped apple and walnuts and vinaigrette dressing*
*Turkey burger on toasted whole-wheat bread*
*Steamed spinach*
*Peach or pear slices topped with vanilla yogurt and*
*1 tablespoon chopped walnuts*
*Decaf iced tea, sparkling water, and/or a glass of wine*

**EVENING AEROBICS/STRESS RELIEF (10 minutes)**

Take a 10 minute after-dinner walk or repeat this morning's Wake-up Stretch and Conditioning routine.

**DRINK A GLASS OF WATER.**

**EVENING BRAIN TRAINING (2 minutes)**

TIP-OF-THE-TONGUE. How did you do today? Check out your list and memorize the connections to store those words in long-term memory.

LOOK, SNAP, CONNECT. Here are more word pairs to learn in order to practice this skill:

globe — wrench
popcorn — crown
clock — lizard

**NIGHTTIME SNACK**

*Fresh fruit*

# DAY 4

**TOTAL TIME INVESTMENT = 36 MINUTES**

## WAKE-UP STRETCH AND CONDITIONING (4 minutes)

STRETCH #3: SITTING TOE TOUCH. Sit on the floor with your legs straight in front of you, ankles almost touching with toes pointing toward ceiling. Raise your arms above your head. Keeping yours arms straight and leading with your fingers and head, slowly lean forward and try to touch your toes. Hold the position for a few seconds and then slowly sit back up. Total: 5 times.

STRETCH #2: SIDE STRETCH (see Day 2). Repeat 5 times.

CONDITIONING EXERCISE #1: RUSSIAN DANCER KNEE LIFTS (see Day 1). Total: 15 per side.

EXTRA CREDIT:
CONDITIONING EXERCISE #2: MARCHING SOLDIER (see Day 3). Total: count of 20.

## DRINK A GLASS OF WATER.

**TIP FOR THE DAY**

Make an effort to listen more attentively and remember one thing your spouse or friend has scheduled today, such as an important meeting or event. Ask them about it in the evening—they'll probably appreciate your remembering that detail.

## BREAKFAST

*Two slices whole-wheat French toast*
*(use 1 whole egg plus 1 egg white) with all-fruit jam*
*½ cup low-fat cottage cheese with ½ cup fresh or frozen blueberries*
*Tea, coffee, water, or sparkling juice*

**MORNING BRAIN TRAINING (3 minutes)**

NAME AND FACE RECALL. Let's recheck your memory for names and faces. What are the names of the people below?

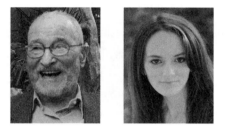

_____   _____

If you don't remember, go back and learn them again. See if you can remember them 15 minutes from now.

Some names suggest a visual image, but you may need to alter the name slightly to conjure up an image. For example, you might see Angela Howe as an *angel* (Angela) hovering over a *house* (Howe). See if you can come up with memorable images for the following names:

**Paul Walling**

**Marina Seigel**

**Olivia Gage**

MEMORY HABITS. At the same time and place as yesterday, check your calendar and plan ahead for the day. Look around so you don't forget something you may need.

EXTRA CREDIT:
STORY METHOD. Think up a story to remember a list of errands.

For example, here is my list for today:

**Get gas for car.**

**Pick up the dry-cleaning.**

**Drop off shoes for repair.**

**Purchase AA batteries.**

To remember my list, I envision myself barefoot (having just dropped my shoes off for repair), filling the car with gas, but the gas spills on my suit jacket. Now I have to take it to the dry cleaners, but they can't clean it unless I get them some AA batteries.

Now create your own list of errands for today and make up a story to remember them.

---

**AEROBICS ON THE GO (12 minutes)**

Spend 10 minutes walking briskly outside or on a treadmill, cycling, or doing an aerobic workout of your choice before starting your day.

OR

Park or get dropped off at least 10 minutes away from your first destination, and walk briskly the rest of the way.

Today, skip the elevator and try taking the stairs two at a time for as many flights as you can (a couple of minutes). I don't recommend this if you're wearing very high heels or have bad knees. If there are no stairs to climb at your destination, spend an extra few minutes doing your initial aerobic workout.

**DRINK A GLASS OF WATER WHEN YOU ARRIVE.**

---

**MIDMORNING SNACK**

*½ cup nonfat yogurt with ½ banana*

**MIDMORNING BRAIN TRAINING (1 minute)**

LOOK, SNAP, CONNECT. Can you remember the word pairs from last night? Here are the first words; try to retrieve your mental images to remember the second word for each pair:

globe _____
popcorn _____
clock _____

**LUNCH**

*2–3 ounces sliced roast beef on rye,*
*with cheddar cheese, lettuce, and tomato (if you like)*
*Iced tea or sparkling water with lemon*

**AFTERNOON STRESS RELIEF (2 minutes)**

Get comfortable and breathe in slowly through your nose. Visualize your breath as it enters your sinuses, flows down into your chest, and expands your rib cage. Slowly breathe out through your nose, following the breath as it rises through your chest and sinuses and finally leaves your body. Repeat for another minute.

**AFTERNOON SNACK**

*Bag of raw vegetables, such as celery, red bell pepper, or carrots*
*1 ounce cheddar cheese*
*Iced tea or water with lemon*

**AFTERNOON BRAIN TRAINING (3 minutes)**

TIP-OF-THE-TONGUE. Here are a few of the tip-of-the tongue challenges that some of my friends have experienced. See if you can use *LOOK, SNAP, CONNECT* so they don't bother you:

1. Who was that wonderful French actor who sang "Thank Heaven, for Little Girls" in the movie *Gigi*? I know I know it. . . .

2. Now I'm blocking on the playwright who wrote *Who's Afraid of Virginia Woolf.* I remember Liz Taylor and Richard Burton in the film, but who wrote that darn play?

3. I was just in Las Vegas, but I can't remember the capital of Nevada. I know it's not Salem, that's Oregon, but what the heck is it?

**DINNER**

*Romaine salad with light Caesar dressing*
*4–6 ounces broiled halibut with salsa*
*½ cup brown rice*
*Steamed broccoli*
*½ banana sliced and drizzled with*
*1 tablespoon chocolate sauce*
*Sparkling water, decaf iced tea, and/or a glass of wine*

**EVENING AEROBICS/STRESS RELIEF (10 minutes)**

Take a 10-minute after-dinner walk or repeat this morning's Wake-Up Stretch and Conditioning routine.

EXTRA CREDIT:
Extend the walk to 15 minutes.

**DRINK A GLASS OF WATER.**

**EVENING BRAIN TRAINING (2 minutes)**

TIP-OF-THE-TONGUE. Here are the answers to my friends' recall delays. Use *LOOK, SNAP, CONNECT* to sear them into your hippocampal memory stores.

*Gigi*—Maurice Chevalier

*Virginia Woolf*—Edward Albee

capital of Nevada—Carson City (try using a snap of Johnny Carson gambling at a casino)

**NIGHTTIME SNACK**
*2–3 cups popcorn, air-popped and without butter*
*(A dash of seasoned salt is fine.)*

**WAKE-UP STRETCH AND CONDITIONING (4 minutes)**

STRETCH #1: SQUAT AND REACH STRETCH (see Day 1). Total: 5 times.

STRETCH #3: SITTING TOE TOUCH (see Day 4). Total: 5 times.

STRETCH #4: CHEST/BACK EXPANDERS. Stand with your feet shoulder width apart, interlace your fingers with palms away from your body, and push your arms straight out in front of you as far as you can. Hold for 2 to 4 seconds, release, and repeat. Now link your hands behind your back. Lift them up slightly, pushing them back and away from your body. Hold for 2 to 4 seconds, release, and repeat. If it is difficult to link your hands behind your back, stretch a rolled towel between them, grabbing each end of the towel. Total: count of 1.

> **TIP FOR THE DAY**
>
> Take a moment to consider what is best to commit to memory, such as people's names, and use your smart phone and other devices for everything else. That way when you see a colleague or acquaintance, the name will roll off your tongue, but if they phone you, you can wish them happy birthday because that information is in your calendar.

CONDITIONING EXERCISE #1: RUSSIAN DANCER KNEE LIFTS (see Day 1). Total: 20 per side.

EXTRA CREDIT:
CONDITIONING EXERCISE #2: MARCHING SOLDIER (see Day 3). Total: count of 20.

CONDITIONING EXERCISE #3: TWISTING PUNCHER. Stand with your feet shoulder width apart, knees slightly bent, and arms at your sides. Begin by twisting to the left and throwing a punch with your right hand toward the upper left corner of the room while pushing up with your right leg. Let your right heel come off the floor while you're punching. Then twist to the right and throw a punch with your left hand at the upper right corner. Total: 5 times per side.

**DRINK A GLASS OF WATER.**

---

**BREAKFAST**

*Orange sections*
*Breakfast burrito:*
*3 egg whites scrambled with*
*1 ounce shredded cheddar cheese and 1 tablespoon salsa*
*and rolled in a warmed corn tortilla*
*Tea, coffee, or sparkling juice*

---

**MORNING BRAIN TRAINING (3 minutes)**

MEMORY HABITS. At the same time and place as yesterday, check your calendar and plan ahead for the day. Look around so you don't forget something you may need.

NAME AND FACE RECALL. Meet Sue Bangel, below. She's an attorney. Spend a few moments to learn her name and face. Here's a hint: Think about her hairstyle and what she does for a living.

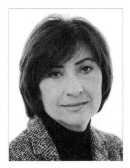

EXTRA CREDIT:
Do the crossword, Sudoku, KenKen, or puzzle of your choice.

**AEROBICS ON THE GO (15 minutes)**

Spend 10 minutes walking briskly outside or on a treadmill, cycling, or doing an aerobic workout of your choice before starting your day. AND
Park or get dropped off at least a few minutes or more away from your first destination and walk briskly the rest of the way.

Skip the elevator and take the stairs for at least one more flight than yesterday. If there are no stairs, increase your initial aerobic workout by a few minutes.

**DRINK A GLASS OF WATER WHEN YOU ARRIVE.**

**MIDMORNING SNACK**

*½ cup nonfat yogurt with 1 tablespoon of raisins mixed in*
*½ apple, sliced and sprinkled with cinnamon*
*Green tea or water*

**MIDMORNING BRAIN TRAINING (2 minutes)**

NAME AND FACE RECALL. Practice your mental prowess in creating visual images for these names that don't immediately bring a snapshot to mind. Your association doesn't have to be exact. For example, you might see Mr. Bakski skiing backward. Try it out on the following names:

**Mr. Monkarsh**

**Mrs. Churchill**

**Dr. Singleton**

**LUNCH**

*Garden vegetable salad with 3–6 ounces diced chicken*
*and vinaigrette dressing*
*Iced tea or sparkling water with lemon*

**AFTERNOON STRESS RELIEF (1 minute)**

Today, do stretch #1 (squat and reach stretch) slowly while breathing normally. Repeat 5 times.

**AFTERNOON SNACK**

*1 cup chicken soup*
*Peach or pear*
*Iced tea or water with lemon*

**AFTERNOON BRAIN TRAINING (3 minutes)**

TIP-OF-THE-TONGUE. Here's some more tip-of-the-tongue fun:

1. I know I know this . . . Who's the guy who wrote *Bonfire of the Vanities*?

2. What's my problem? I can't think of the former name of Thailand; I know it starts with an S.

3. Okay, it's right on the tip of my tongue . . . the name of the newscaster Katie Couric replaced on the evening news.

NAME AND FACE RECALL. Can you recall any of the three names you worked on this morning? If you can't, here are a few clues: I recall seeing a monkey in a car crash, a church on a hill, and a single one-ton weight.

**DINNER**

*Tomato, avocado and sweet onion salad drizzled*
*with olive oil and vinegar*
*4–6-ounces grilled salmon steak with herbs*
*Steamed broccoli*
*½ cup brown rice*
*Fruit sorbet*
*Sparkling water, decaf iced tea, water, and/or a glass of wine*

**EVENING AEROBICS/STRESS RELIEF (10 minutes)**

Take a 10-minute after-dinner walk or repeat this morning's Wake-Up Stretch and Conditioning routine.

**DRINK A GLASS OF WATER.**

**EVENING BRAIN TRAINING (1 minute)**

NAME AND FACE RECALL. Do you remember this woman's name?

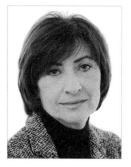

**NIGHTTIME SNACK**

*Frozen fruit-juice bar*

**WAKE-UP STRETCH AND CONDITIONING (6 minutes)**

STRETCH #1: SQUAT AND REACH STRETCH (see Day 1). Total: 5 times.

STRETCH #2: SIDE STRETCH (see Day 2). Total: 5 per side.

STRETCH #4: CHEST/BACK EXPANDERS (see Day 5). Repeat 4 times.

CONDITIONING EXERCISE #1: RUSSIAN DANCER KNEE LIFTS (see Day 1). Repeat 20 times.

EXTRA CREDIT:
CONDITIONING EXERCISE #2: MARCHING SOLDIER (see Day 3). Total: count of 20.

CONDITIONING EXERCISE #3: TWISTING PUNCHER (see Day 5). Total: 10 per side.

**DRINK A GLASS OF WATER.**

**BREAKFAST**

*½ grapefruit*
*Open-face egg-white sandwich*
*(2 cooked egg whites on 1 slice sourdough toast*
*with 1 ounce cheddar cheese and a slice of tomato)*
*Tea, coffee, or water*

## TIP FOR THE DAY

A major source of stress is clutter and disorganization. Try to spend at least 15 minutes today decluttering and organizing one specific but important place you use each day—it could be your bulletin board, desk, or a closet. Be realistic about how much you can accomplish in the time that you have. You're better off organizing just one part of your bulletin board and leaving the rest for later than feeling stressed out that you couldn't declutter the entire board. Notice how great it feels to get rid of unnecessary clutter.

**MORNING BRAIN TRAINING (4 minutes)**

MEMORY HABITS. At the same time and place as yesterday, check your calendar and plan ahead for the day. Look around so you don't forget something you may need.

TIP-OF-THE-TONGUE. How did it go with yesterday's questions? Here's the first answer, along with a clue to never forget it again:

*Bonfire of the Vanities*—**Tom Wolfe (see a wolf sitting at her vanity table with a bonfire blazing outside the window)**

Here are the other two answers. See if you can come up with a way to link these word pairs to keep them in your memory forever.

**Thailand—Siam**

**evening newscaster—Dan Rather**

NAME AND FACE RECALL. I want you to meet Barry Stuberman. Use *LOOK, SNAP, CONNECT* to memorize his name and face. Clue: Look for a memorable facial feature that perhaps sounds like his name. The memory aid doesn't have to be exact—just close enough to jog your recall later.

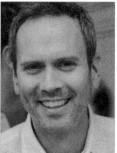

EXTRA CREDIT:
Do the crossword, Sudoku, KenKen, or puzzle of your choice.

## AEROBICS ON THE GO (15 minutes)

Spend 15 minutes on a morning walk, treadmill, bicycle, or do a workout of your choice.

AND

Park or get dropped off at least a 5-minute walk from your first destination. Walk briskly the rest of the way.

Skip the elevator and take the stairs—try to add an extra flight. If there are no stairs, increase your initial aerobic workout by a few minutes.

EXTRA CREDIT:

Increase your aerobics session to 30 minutes.

## DRINK A GLASS OF WATER WHEN YOU ARRIVE.

## MIDMORNING SNACK

*½ apple, sliced and sprinkled with cinnamon*
*½ cup low-fat cottage cheese*
*Green tea or water*

## MIDMORNING BRAIN TRAINING (3 minutes)

STORY METHOD AND CHUNKING. You can use the story method along with chunking (grouping items together) to remember practical information such as your license plate number. One of my old cars had the following license plate number:

# 2 Y S L 7 6 T

Here is how I remembered it: I visualized the designer, Yves Saint Laurent, walking with his imaginary twin brother (2 YSLs); they come across a marching band playing "76 Trombones."

Now check out your license plate number or your driver's license number and see how creative you can be with the Story Method and Chunking.

---

**LUNCH**

*2–3 ounces sliced turkey in a sandwich, with*
*1 ounce Swiss cheese, mustard, lettuce, and tomato (if you wish)*
*Grapes*
*Iced tea or sparkling water with lemon*

---

**AFTERNOON STRESS RELIEF (5 minutes)**

Take a walk or have a conversation with a friend or do both if possible. Just make sure that you break away from work for at least 5 minutes. Avoid online shopping or entertainment or tasks that might cause stress. This break should be purely relaxing and away from your usual work mode and daily routine.

---

**AFTERNOON SNACK**

*Sliced raw vegetables*
*1 ounce almonds (about 2 dozen)*
*Iced tea or water with lemon*

---

**AFTERNOON BRAIN TRAINING (3 minutes)**

STORY METHOD AND CHUNKING. Do you remember your driver's license or license plate number? Do you remember my old license plate number?

MEMORY PLACES. Take inventory of your memory places. How are your current ones working? Can you add some new ones? Are you having less trouble remembering where you put things?

**DINNER**

> *Arugula and shredded Parmesan cheese salad tossed in*
> *balsamic vinegar and olive oil dressing*
> *4–6 ounces sliced chicken breast with fettuccine and tomato sauce*
> *Zucchini rounds pan-fried in olive oil with garlic*
> *Sliced strawberries (may be drizzled with 1 teaspoon chocolate sauce)*
> *Sparkling water, decaf iced tea, water, and/or a glass of wine*

**EVENING AEROBICS/STRESS RELIEF (10 minutes)**

Take a 10-minute after-dinner walk or repeat this morning's Wake-up Stretch and Conditioning routine.

EXTRA CREDIT:
Extend your walk to 15 minutes.

**DRINK A GLASS OF WATER.**

**EVENING BRAIN TRAINING (1 minute)**

NAME AND FACE RECALL. Do you remember the guy you met earlier today?

Yes, it's Barry Stuberman. I could never forget his name because he has a stubbly beard and he is a man (Stuberman). If he ever shaves his beard, we'll need to come up with another memory cue, of course.

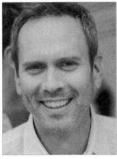

**NIGHTTIME SNACK**

> *2–3 cups popcorn (air popped, no butter)*

**WAKE-UP STRETCH AND CONDITIONING (6 minutes)**

STRETCH #1: SQUAT AND REACH STRETCH. Total: 5 times.

STRETCH #2: SIDE STRETCH. 5 per side.

STRETCH #3: SITTING TOE TOUCH. Total: count of 5.

STRETCH #4: CHEST/BACK EXPANDERS (see Day 5). Total: count of 4.

CONDITIONING EXERCISE #1: RUSSIAN DANCER KNEE LIFTS. Total: 20 per side.

EXTRA CREDIT:
CONDITIONING EXERCISE #2: MARCHING SOLDIER. Total: count of 30.

CONDITIONING EXERCISE #3: TWISTING PUNCHER. Total: 5 per side.

CONDITIONING EXERCISE #4: STANDING CRUNCHES. Stand straight with your feet slightly apart. Lift your arms straight overhead, palms facing each other and hands fisted. Take a deep breath. Exhale as you lift your right knee and pull your arms down powerfully, as if there were weights in your fists, bending at the elbow. Inhale as your arms go back up, and repeat with your left knee. Keep your stomach pulled in and tight, especially as you exhale. Total: count of 10.

**DRINK A GLASS OF WATER.**

**BREAKFAST**

*Toasted bagel with low-fat cream cheese and 1 slice smoked salmon;*
*add tomato and onion as desired*
*Mixed berries*
*Tea, coffee, water, or sparkling juice*

**MORNING BRAIN TRAINING (3 minutes)**

MEMORY HABITS. Make your daily checks as you do each morning.

ABSTRACT WORD PAIRS. Let's ratchet up your word pair power by trying *LOOK, SNAP, CONNECT* to link more abstract words together. Since these words don't readily lead to a visual image, you'll have to be more creative to come up with a snapshot in your mind. For instance, for a word such as *idea,* you might visualize a lightbulb; for *clause,* you might see Santa Claus:

ornate — asylum

opaque — childproof

ornery — ephemeral

infer — adopt

EXTRA CREDIT:
Do the crossword, Sudoku, KenKen, or puzzle of your choice.

**AEROBICS ON THE GO (25 minutes)**

Spend 15 minutes on a morning walk, treadmill, or bicycle or do a workout of your choice.

AND

Park or get dropped off at least a 5-minute walk from your first destination, and walk briskly the rest of the way.

Skip the elevator and take the stairs and continue to gradually increase the number of stairs each day. If there are no stairs, increase your initial aerobic workout by a few minutes.

EXTRA CREDIT:
Extend your walk to 30 minutes.

**DRINK A GLASS OF WATER WHEN YOU ARRIVE.**

---

**MIDMORNING SNACK**

*Hard-boiled egg (or whites of 3 hard-boiled eggs)*
*1 cup soup of your choice*
*Green tea or water*

---

**MIDMORNING BRAIN TRAINING (4 minutes)**

To improve your attention, do a 1-minute relaxation exercise. Close your eyes and breathe slowly to put yourself into a mindful state. Ideally, do this when you're alone so you won't be distracted.

LEARNING COMPLEX NAMES. It can be a challenge to create name snaps for long or complex names, but you can break up the syllables and link up word snaps for the syllables in names in order to remember them better. For example, to remember Mr. Schindler, you might visualize a shin in a lair. Movie fans will probably bypass this strategy by thinking of the movie about his list. For Mrs. Weinkauf, you might see her coughing after sipping her wine. Try this approach on these names:

Marcia Salazar

Marcus Delman

Annette Runyan

---

**LUNCH**

*Salad Niçoise:*
*(butter lettuce with tuna, green beans, tomatoes, olives, egg whites,*
*bell pepper, and artichoke hearts, tossed in olive oil and vinegar dressing)*
*Iced tea or sparkling water with lemon*

---

**AFTERNOON STRESS RELIEF (5 minutes)**

Take a 5-minute break to do any stress-relief exercise of your choosing.

---

**AFTERNOON SNACK**

*Guacamole*
*(½ avocado, mashed, with 1 tablespoon light mayonnaise,*
*¼ cup drained salsa, and lemon juice to taste)*
*Fresh vegetable sticks*
*Iced tea or water with lemon*

---

**AFTERNOON BRAIN TRAINING (2 minutes)**

ABSTRACT WORD PAIRS. See how many of this morning's word pairs you can remember:

ornate _____

opaque _____

ornery _____

infer _____

---

---

**DINNER**

*Spinach salad with chopped apple and walnuts,*
*drizzled with vinegar and olive oil*
*4–6 ounces grilled sirloin steak or chicken*
*½ baked potato*
*½ cup of frozen yogurt*
*Sparkling water, decaf iced tea, water, and/or a glass of wine*

---

**EVENING AEROBICS/STRESS RELIEF (10 minutes)**

Take a 10-minute after-dinner walk or repeat this morning's Wake-up Stretch and Conditioning routine.

EXTRA CREDIT:
Extend your walk to 15 minutes.

**DRINK A GLASS OF WATER.**

---

**EVENING BRAIN TRAINING (2 minutes)**

NAME RECALL. Do you remember the more complex names you taught yourself earlier today? To help you, below are the first names. See if you can come up with the last names:

Marcia _____

Marcus _____

Annette _____

---

**NIGHTTIME SNACK**

*Fresh or frozen mixed berries*

---

Congratulations! You have just completed the first week of your Alzheimer's prevention program. Each day, you should be feeling more confident about your memory performance, ability to deal with stress, and increasing physical stamina. Continue to use the strategies you've learned and modify them as needed as they become your new healthy lifestyle habits. During the weeks, months, and years ahead, you will continue to enjoy these rewards if you stick with your program, and you'll feel great knowing that you're doing all you can now to protect your brain for the future. If you keep going with the program, and I hope you will, be creative with the exercises. In the next chapter you can retest yourself to see how your scores have improved.

"WE ARE WHAT WE
REPEATEDLY DO.
EXCELLENCE, THEREFORE,
IS NOT AN ACT BUT
A HABIT."

—ARISTOTLE

# Protecting Your Brain for Life

I WAS AT AN AIRPORT NEWSSTAND, WAITING IN LINE to buy a magazine. A woman in her mid-60s standing behind me tapped me on the shoulder and said, "Dr. Small, do you remember me?"

I usually dread that question, but this time I immediately recalled both her face and her name. How could I forget Jessie B.? She was one of the earliest volunteers in our Alzheimer's prevention study. She had been concerned about her memory because several times she had gone to the market for something, gotten distracted while shopping, and come home having forgotten the item she went for. After participating in our program for a few weeks, she enjoyed dramatic improvements in her everyday memory skills, short-term recall, and general mental focus.

"Hello, Jessie," I said. "How are you?"

"Dr. Small, you'd be proud of me." She grinned. "I'm still looking, snapping, and connecting, and my memory is as strong as ever."

We chatted a bit about how she'd stuck with her healthy brain lifestyle over the years and how her worry about her family history of Alzheimer's disease kept her motivated. She looked down and said, "I did fall off the wagon a few times, though. You know, sometimes when my kids stressed me out, or my late-night cookie binges got the best of me, but I was able to forgive myself and get back on my program." She described several strategies that helped her, including a diary she kept in which she charted her progress each day.

I suddenly realized I had to hurry to catch my flight, so we said our good-byes. As I was rushing toward my gate, I heard her shout after me, "Dr. Small, you forgot your magazine." Nobody's perfect.

Every day, you wake up with another chance to protect your brain from Alzheimer's disease. Even if you weren't able to reach all your goals yesterday—perhaps you didn't exercise or maybe you over did it on dessert—there's no reason to despair. It's easy to get right back on track for the long haul, just as Jessie did. It's the day-to-day cumulative effect of a lifetime of preventive strategies that gives the Alzheimer's prevention program its power.

## Objective Recall Checkup

To see how much you have already improved your memory, use the following objective recall assessment and compare your results to the first one you did in Chapter 2. Here is a list of 10 unrelated words similar to those you memorized before you started the program. To determine your current Objective Recall score, set the timer for 1 minute and in that time try to memorize the following word list:

## OBJECTIVE RECALL ASSESSMENT

shark

radio

eel

city

locker

ivy

lizard

giraffe

road

chopsticks

ice

After the minute, reset the timer for 10 minutes and do something else. When the timer alerts you, write down as many of the words as you can remember without looking back at the list.

Now go back to Chapter 2 and look up your baseline score. How much better is your score now? 1 point? 2 points? 3 or more? If you did the exercises, you're likely to see improvement. That is what we have found in our studies involving thousands of people who have gotten serious about protecting their brains through Alzheimer's prevention strategies. If you don't see much improvement yet, give yourself more time so that the exercises can take effect. Everyone learns at his own pace. Stick to the program and repeat your Objective Recall assessment in a week or two. Even though this kind of exercise may not seem directly related to your particular memory concerns, it can help with a variety of challenges.

The first seven days of your program are just the beginning. You've probably already shown yourself that you can improve your memory skills in that brief time. You're also beginning to form new habits and getting used to your healthy brain lifestyle. You may have lost a pound or two with the Alzheimer's prevention diet, and perhaps you're feeling more energy and sleeping better thanks to your new aerobics routine.

But we're all human, and this chapter will help you continue your program even if you find yourself slipping back to your old lifestyle habits once in a while. The important thing is to keep protecting your brain for the rest of your life.

## Knowing Why Helps

Understanding how behavior influences brain and body fitness, both now and in the future, motivates people to initiate and maintain healthy lifestyle habits. Dr. Catherine Sarkisian and colleagues at UCLA enrolled a group of sedentary older adults in a walking exercise program that also included education on the health benefits of their exercise. After seven weeks, the research volunteers were walking more on their own than they did before the intervention. The volunteers also reported improved mental health and quality of life. They claimed to experience less pain, higher energy levels, and better sleep.

We haven't completed all our studies on why the Alzheimer's prevention program appears to be so effective. It's possible that the exercises directly protect our brains against the disease, or they may have an indirect effect by reducing the risks for other diseases, such as diabetes, that are associated with Alzheimer's. Either way, our brains benefit.

As you continue your prevention program beyond the first week, keep in mind some of the connections between your everyday lifestyle choices and their effects on your brain health:

- Brain aging and the buildup of plaques and tangles begin decades before any symptoms of Alzheimer's disease are obvious, so it's never too early (or too late) to start protecting your brain.
- Genetics accounts for only part of your risk for Alzheimer's

disease. Even if you have a genetic risk, your lifestyle still has an important impact on maintaining your brain health.

- Inflammation accelerates brain aging, so keep up your physical exercise program, eat omega-3 fats, get enough sleep, and take other actions to control chronic inflammation.
- Combining several Alzheimer's prevention strategies has a synergistic effect on brain function and memory ability, and these benefits can be immediate as well as long-term.

## Don't Forget to Use Your Memory Tools

Memory strategies similar to *LOOK, SNAP, CONNECT* can improve everyday memory ability, and with practice these methods will become second nature. Here are a few things to keep in mind to help us through some of the more common memory challenges.

### Names and Faces

- When you meet someone, look for a striking facial feature to create a face snap. Think about what the person's name sounds like or means, and create a name snap that you can picture in your mind to connect it to the face snap.
- When you first meet someone, try to repeat their name and ask specific questions about their life.

### Where We Put Things

- Park your car in the same area every day or use *LOOK, SNAP, CONNECT* to remember where you parked. For example, if you park in section 2D, create a mental snapshot of *two* large, scary *dogs* sitting on top of your car. I don't think I would forget that.
- Create memory places in your house or office for your keys, glasses, phone, and other often misplaced objects.
- When you travel, be mindful about where you put things by creating temporary memory places in your room.

### What We Plan to Do

- Before leaving home, think ahead about your plans for the day. Check your calendar so you don't overlook an appointment or something you need for the day.
- Create this memory habit by doing it at the same time and place each day.

### Tip-of-the-Tongue Phenomena

- Jot down your associations to the word or phrase you are searching for.
- If the word comes to you later, write it down next to your associations. Otherwise, look it up or ask someone.
- Use *LOOK, SNAP, CONNECT* to link the word or phrase to your associations.

# Physical Fitness

Of all the lifestyle habits that may protect your brain health, the scientific evidence is most compelling for the effects of regular physical conditioning. Recent research shows that people who engage in moderate physical activity have a 40 percent lower risk for developing Alzheimer's disease. Keep in mind the following points to maintain your healthy brain athletic program:

- You don't have to become a triathlete to get enough physical exercise to protect your brain. Set reasonable and attainable goals, such as 15 to 30 minutes of brisk walking daily.
- Strength and resistance training not only build muscle mass and protect bones and joints; they can also improve memory and brain function.
- Maintaining balance and stability helps people avoid injuries that can lead to cognitive decline.

- Find an exercise routine that is fun and challenging; that way you'll want to keep it up for the long run.
- If you have a busy lifestyle, try to work your exercise into your daily routine and take note of how you feel while exercising. Consider walking faster so you can feel your heart rate rise a bit more.

## Staying Sharp with Mental Workouts

Engaging in mentally stimulating activities will fire up your neural circuits and train your brain to perform better. When considering mental workouts, keep the following in mind:

- Your goal is to train but not strain your brain—find brain games that are fun and stimulating but not so difficult that you want to give up.
- Cross train your brain by alternating right-brain visual games with left-brain verbal puzzles.
- Use computer technology to exercise your mind and improve cognitive skills.
- Stay socially connected—engaging conversations with friends do more for cognitive skills than watching TV does.

## Stress Management

Chronic stress causes wear and tear on our neural circuits and often contributes to cognitive impairment as we age. We can't eliminate all the stress from our lives, but we can learn to manage it in a way that protects our brain health:

- Getting a good night's sleep reduces chronic inflammation, improves memory, and makes us more resilient when dealing with stressful events.
- Minimizing multitasking with your gadgets can improve mental focus and lower stress levels. Try to balance your technology time with off-line time.

- Take breaks throughout the day for meditation, breathing exercises, and other strategies to reduce stress.
- Get realistic about how much work you take on and plan ahead to eliminate sources of stress that you can control. Try delegating tasks and cutting out unnecessary ones.

# The Alzheimer's Prevention Diet

Recent studies provide a guide on healthy brain nutrition choices that may lower your risk for Alzheimer's disease. As you build on your first week of the Alzheimer's prevention program, consider the following:

- Complex carbohydrates and whole grains are brain protective.
- Daydreaming about eating unhealthy snacks actually satisfies the urge for those snacks.
- Try eating fish twice a week to get enough omega-3 fats to protect brain health and stabilize mood. Avoid fish high in mercury, for example shark and swordfish.
- Keep your brain healthy with antioxidant fruits and vegetables, as well as protein from poultry, fish, and soybeans.
- Some alcohol and caffeine may protect the brain, but don't overdo it. If you're going to drink either one, do it in moderation.

# Become Partners with Your Doctor

Learn as much as you can about your own health and health care options and develop a partnership with your doctor to help you make reasonable health care choices. Investigators at the University of Pittsburgh found that when doctors advise their patients about healthy lifestyle behaviors, the patients are more likely to follow through and engage in healthier behaviors, resulting in better weight control and other positive health outcomes than patients who don't receive such advice.

Consider the following to empower yourself to protect your brain more effectively:

- Be proactive with your doctors and designate one of them as your primary physician. Be sure to review *all* your health concerns, medications, and questions with your primary doctor, and keep no secrets—especially about any memory issues.
- Follow your doctor's advice in treating physical illnesses such as hypertension or diabetes, which can put your brain at risk when left untreated.
- Be careful about medication side effects and remember to include over-the-counter drugs and dietary supplements when discussing side effects with your doctor.
- Vitamins and supplements offer promise as brain-protective strategies, but don't substitute supplements for a healthy brain diet.

## If at First You Don't Succeed

Whether your healthy lifestyle program focuses on losing weight or on increasing the size of your frontal lobe, a personalized Alzheimer's prevention program usually comes down to self-discipline. Doctors, trainers, and coaches can help drive us forward to reach our goals, but we need to be compassionate toward ourselves if we falter now and then.

Research shows that compassion for ourselves is, in fact, more effective at helping us get back on our programs sooner and stay on them for the long haul than constantly reprimanding ourselves for our mistakes and feeling guilty about them. Drs. Claire Adams of Louisiana State University and Mark Leary of Duke University studied college women who participated in a weight-loss program. Those women who were taught to think compassionately about their eating—to forgive themselves if they overate—experienced less stress and actually ate less during the study. The investigators believe that people who were too hard on themselves if they fell off their diet ate more in order to cope with those feelings. When we give ourselves permission to enjoy an occasional "cheat eat," we end up eating less in the long run.

You'll notice that the first seven days of the Alzheimer's prevention program offer some alternatives. It's not intended to be rigid. The fear that omitting one exercise or missing one day will lead to a lifetime of self-indulgence is a distortion. Try focusing on the positive—the things you have accomplished. The bottom line is, don't beat yourself up for not being perfect. It's human to make mistakes, but it's also helpful to quickly get back to your Alzheimer's prevention program so you can begin noticing the benefits again. Systematic research has found that when people gain confidence in their ability to make positive changes in their behaviors, that confidence translates into real change and healthier lifestyle habits.

I've always enjoyed drawing graphs, charts, and diagrams. When I was a kid my sisters would tease me about being a math and science geek, but seeing a visual image often had a greater impact on my understanding of things than just words, not unlike how creating visual snapshots of memories can make them more rememberable.

I recommend that you keep track of your progress as you continue working through your program over the coming weeks and months. Research on self-monitoring shows that it does have a significant impact on the success of a healthy lifestyle program. Each of us needs to find the form of self-monitoring that works best for our individual preferences and lifestyles. For someone on a diet, monitoring can be as simple as standing on a reliable scale every week at the same time, while others find that it's how their jeans fit that gives them the information they seek.

Some people like to plot their progress on charts; others use diaries. You can use these and other monitoring systems to encourage yourself in areas of strength and to help you focus more in areas that need additional work. Here are some examples from two of our volunteers.

**Q: I have a history of Alzheimer's in my family, and I'd like to get involved in a research study. How do I go about doing that?**

**A:** It's great that you want to volunteer for a study. Our group at UCLA is always looking for volunteers, and you can reach us at www.longevity.ucla.edu. The national Alzheimer's Association (www.alz.org) and the National Institutes of Health (www.clinicaltrials.gov) also provide listings at a national level. Other opportunities are available at local university medical centers.

Steve C. kept up with all the new research about brain health and memory fitness and was serious about trying the Alzheimer's prevention program. After his baseline assessment, he realized that his biggest challenge was to find time to exercise and relax, so he decided to graph his daily progress in those two areas. He planned to focus on walking for his aerobic conditioning and meditation for stress reduction. He plotted the time he spent in minutes each day doing each one.

When he reviewed his week, Steve quickly realized that he was on track Monday and Tuesday but by midweek he dropped the ball. Wednesday was when he had an all-day marketing conference. He did pick things up as the week went on and made up for lost time over the weekend. In the future, he decided to plan ahead if he had conferences to make sure he got in enough time for his workout.

Jessie B., our volunteer who got anxious about her age-related memory changes when she forgot to buy certain items at the market, didn't like charts and graphs. She preferred to follow her progress by keeping a diary in a daily calendar. She wrote in comments to cheer

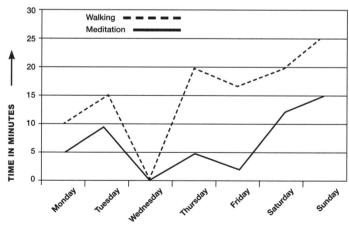

## STEVE'S DAILY EXERCISES

## JESSIE'S CALENDAR

**May 2**
Tuesday

| APRIL | | | | | | | | JUNE | | | | | | |
|---|---|---|---|---|---|---|---|---|---|---|---|---|---|---|
| S | M | T | W | T | F | S | | S | M | T | W | T | F | S |
| | | | | | 1 | 2 | | 1 | 2 | 3 | 4 | 5 | 6 | 7 |
| 3 | 4 | 5 | 6 | 7 | 8 | 9 | | 8 | 9 | 10 | 11 | 12 | 13 | 14 |
| 10 | 11 | 12 | 13 | 14 | 15 | 16 | | 15 | 16 | 17 | 18 | 19 | 20 | 21 |
| 17 | 18 | 19 | 20 | 21 | 22 | 23 | | 22 | 23 | 24 | 25 | 26 | 27 | 28 |
| 24 | 25 | 26 | 27 | 28 | 29 | 30 | | 29 | 30 | 31 | | | | |

|  |  |
|---|---|
| 8:00 | Breakfast: egg-white omelet, green tea, blueberries (Dr. Small would be proud.) |
| 9:00 | Parked my car at a distance—5-minute walk . . . YES!!! |
| 10:00 | My daughter called for money again. Okay, so I ate two donuts. |
| 11:00 | Took a 10-minute meditation break. Feeling better already. |
| 12:00 | Grilled chicken sandwich for lunch—you go girl . . . you're back on track. |
| 1:00 | |
| 2:00 | Took a break to do a Sudoku puzzle—finished it in 10 minutes! |
| 3:00 | I'm starving and would love those chips but I grabbed a yogurt and raisins instead. |
| 4:00 | Did some more brain games; practiced "look, snap, connect." |
| 5:00 | Called daughter—we're all calmer now. Offered to take her out to dinner. |
| 6:00 | |
| 7:00 | Dinner went well; we had a few laughs and I stuck to my diet: tomato sea bass, steamed spinach, and NO potatoes (ouch—that was hard to resist). |
| 8:00 | 1 glass of water |
| 9:00 | Brushed teeth early to avoid snacks; turned off TV and read my book. |

herself along when she met a goal and push herself harder if she fell short.

In the next few weeks, as you continue to build your healthy brain habits, try charting your progress. You might want to fill in some of the blank graphs in Appendix 1, begin a health-tracking program on your smart phone, or use whatever self-monitoring approach works best for you. You can also return to Chapter 2 and gauge your progress by using the assessment questionnaires. See how much better you're doing in each of the areas of your program. If you haven't reached your goals yet, be patient with yourself and continue on with your program.

## Keep Your Brain Healthy for Good

If we take charge of our everyday lifestyle choices, we can push back the age at which Alzheimer's symptoms might begin—perhaps by several years, which in some cases can mean for the rest of our lives. Even if scientists one day come up with a miracle drug that can cure dementia, it will always be easier to protect healthy brain cells than to try to repair damaged ones. For now, prevention is the key to protecting our brains.

We know that genetics is not the whole story when it comes to the onset of Alzheimer's disease. Physical conditioning, healthy diet, mental exercise, and stress management can make a difference in how we feel and function now and in the future. Add ongoing social engagement, effective medical management, and a routine that makes it easy to integrate these strategies into your daily life and you have a perfect prescription for an Alzheimer's prevention program.

"WHY IS IT THAT OUR MEMORY
IS GOOD ENOUGH TO RETAIN
THE LEAST TRIVIALITY THAT
HAPPENS TO US, AND YET NOT
GOOD ENOUGH TO RECOLLECT
HOW OFTEN WE HAVE TOLD IT
TO THE SAME PERSON?"

—FRANÇOIS DE LA ROCHEFOUCAULD
(1613—1680)

# New
# Resources

SINCE THE INITIAL publication of *The Alzheimer's Prevention Program*, new research has dominated the headlines. Readers across the country have been asking me questions about these new studies, particularly how the findings might apply to their own Alzheimer's prevention programs.

In this section, I want to answer some of my most frequently asked questions. I've also thrown in some new brain teasers and additional resources, websites, and tips to enhance your program.

# Frequently Asked Questions

Q: **Is it true that a new cancer drug is being tested as an Alzheimer's disease treatment?**

A: Yes. So far, the tests have been performed only on mice. Cancer drugs generally work by preventing the growth of abnormal cancer cells. University of Pennsylvania scientists are testing a drug called EpoD (short for epothilone D) that was developed to treat cancer because the compound *over* stabilizes the tiny tubules necessary for cancer cells to divide and proliferate—meaning the cancer does not grow or increase. Also, EpoD can penetrate the brain at relatively low doses that don't cause side effects. The scientists realized that this ability to strengthen microtubules might help vulnerable brain cells in Alzheimer's disease by fortifying the microtubules that comprise the misfolded proteins of tau tangles in an Alzheimer's brain. The mice the scientists used in their tests had a human Alzheimer's gene, which impaired their cognition—the animals tended to get lost when crawling through a maze that should have been familiar.

As predicted, EpoD stopped further brain buildup of tau tangles, and the mice were less forgetful when wandering through their mazes. The drug has not yet been tested in humans nor has it been approved as a cancer treatment so, even though these initial results are promising, it may be years before we know if EpoD will be effective for patients with Alzheimer's dementia or those at risk for developing the disease.

Q: **I heard that some scientists discovered that Alzheimer's spreads through the brain like an infection. Should I be worried about catching the disease from someone who has it?**

A: Swedish scientists from Linköping University reported that toxic proteins are transferred from brain cell to brain cell, but you have no need to worry about being infected by an Alzheimer's disease bug. This is not an infection like a cold or pneumonia but a spread of cellular dysfunction from cell to cell within an affected brain. For many years, scientists have known that the disease spreads through the brain in a characteristic pattern expanding through the cortex, the outer rim of cells that control most mental abilities, but this research was the first time that the process was depicted at the cellular level. In laboratory experiments, the researchers showed that a sick brain cell could "infect" other cells nearby. Because this breakthrough study helps scientists understand how

Alzheimer's progresses, it offers an opportunity to develop new treatments to stop the spread of the disease throughout the brain.

Q: **A coworker told me that diabetes doubles the risk for getting Alzheimer's disease. I've had diabetes for years. Should I be worried about developing Alzheimer's?**

A: A large-scale Japanese study showed that people who had diabetes were twice as likely to develop Alzheimer's disease and had a greater risk for any form of dementia. To confirm the suspected connection between diabetes and dementia, investigators from Kyushu University followed 1,000 volunteers for 15 years. Of the 230 research subjects who developed dementia, those who had diabetes had a 74 percent higher risk of developing dementia either from Alzheimer's, small strokes in the brain, or some other cause. The scientists found that the odds of subjects with diabetes getting Alzheimer's disease was about double compared to the subjects who did not have diabetes.

Precisely how diabetes leads to Alzheimer's and other dementias is not certain—it could result from small strokes in the brain known as microvascular changes, decreased blood flow, or inability of brain cells to get enough glucose, which is a primary problem in diabetes. The body becomes resistant to the effects of insulin, the hormone that transports glucose from the blood into cells.

Two of the key Alzheimer's prevention strategies—physical exercise and healthy nutrition—are known to prevent diabetes and improve symptoms of the disease. Getting started and remaining on an Alzheimer's prevention program will help your body fight off diabetes and increase the likelihood that you will stave off symptoms of Alzheimer's disease as well.

Q: **Is it true that air pollution can speed up mental decline and even increase small strokes in the brain?**

A: A recent study from Brown University demonstrated an association between short-term exposure to air pollution (at levels considered safe) and an increased risk for a stroke. Long-term exposure was associated with faster cognitive decline. The heightened risk for a stroke occurred within 12 to 14 hours of exposure, and it was associated with pollution from automobile traffic in particular. These findings suggest that avoiding exposure to smog is another way to maintain brain health and avoid cognitive decline.

THE ALZHEIMER'S PREVENTION PROGRAM

Q: **I read somewhere that eating fish can make your brain larger. Is that possible?**

A: It's true—fish eaters have larger brains, and, in general, a bigger brain is a better brain, especially when volume is preserved in areas controlling cognition. Researchers at the University of Pittsburgh performed MRI brain scans on 260 volunteers who had been followed for 10 years. They found that those who ate fish regularly had less shrinkage in areas of their brains controlling memory compared with volunteers who did not eat much fish. Regular fish eaters also had a lower risk for developing mild cognitive impairment or Alzheimer's disease. The subjects with bigger brains ate fish between one to four times each week.

Scientists are not exactly sure how fish preserves brain size and health, but they describe some interesting theories. The omega-3 fatty acids in fish likely protect the brain from neuronal destruction due to inflammation and oxidation. Omega-3 fats have anti-inflammatory effects that counteract the neuron-destructive brain inflammation that results from aging, being overweight, or avoiding regular exercise. These brain-protective fats also fight oxidative stress that causes wear and tear on our brain cells as we age. Study volunteers who ate fried fish rather than grilled or baked fish had smaller brains and higher risks for memory decline—this is not surprising since fried fish does not have a high concentration of omega-3 fats.

Fish lovers often worry about eating too much fish, and most authorities recommend eating it only twice a week due to concern about mercury exposure. However, avoiding swordfish, shark, and other large predatory fish will lower your chances of ingesting too much mercury. Also, don't forget that tilapia is a fish to skip if you want your omega-3 benefits. For people who don't like fish, an omega-3 supplement is a good idea. I recommend 1,000 milligrams each day, and make sure it contains brain-protective docosahexaenoic acid or DHA.

Q: **I saw on TV that doctors had used electric probes to stimulate the brain and it improved memory and symptoms of Alzheimer's. Is it like electroshock therapy and is it dangerous?**

A: In a small study of five Alzheimer's patients with mild dementia, electrical stimulators were implanted in brain memory centers. To power the stimulators, pacemaker-sized battery packs were implanted under the skin of each patient's chest. After a year, the scientists found that the patients' brain memory centers were functioning better as measured by PET scans, and the brain function improvement correlated with better memory scores. The findings are encouraging but need to be repeated in a larger group of patients. Although the patients tolerated the treatment well, scientists are now studying less invasive ways to stimulate these same brain memory centers, through electrodes placed on the scalp, rather than implanted surgically.

Q: **Everyone is talking about an impending Alzheimer's epidemic. What's going to happen in the next few decades? Are we going to become a nation of demented baby boomers?**

A: In March of 2012, the Alzheimer's Association reported that here in the U.S. we're spending $200 billion each year caring for Alzheimer's victims. As 80 million U.S. baby boomers start reaching age 65, their risk for the disease grows. By 2050, we can expect more than 100 million Alzheimer's patients worldwide if we do nothing to fight the disease. Another frightening revelation was that one out of every seven Alzheimer's patients lives alone. By definition, patients with dementia cannot take care of themselves and need help from others.

This crisis led President Obama to sign the National Alzheimer's Project Act to accelerate research, education, and caregiving efforts. Large-scale drug prevention trials are already underway, but it will take years for these studies to yield results. Scientists at the University of California, San Francisco, have concluded that up to half of Alzheimer's cases are potentially attributable to risk factors under our own control. They estimated that if we could reduce modifiable risk factors (e.g., stop smoking, start exercising, lose weight) by 25 percent, we could potentially prevent as many as 500,000 cases of Alzheimer's in the U.S. and 3 million worldwide. While we're waiting for science to catch up, there's no reason not to do everything we can to protect our brain health. An Alzheimer's prevention program will improve your memory ability right away and likely delay the onset of Alzheimer's symptoms in the future.

Q: **I have been tested and found out I have a genetic risk for Alzheimer's disease. Should I even bother starting a prevention program? I mean, what's the use?**

A: Having a genetic risk for Alzheimer's disease is no reason to give up on your brain health—genetic factors only account for part of the risk. Scientists at Washington University in St. Louis found that even people with the APOE-4 genetic risk for Alzheimer's disease have control over their brain aging. *Only*

20 percent of the population who are APOE-4 carriers are more likely to get Alzheimer's symptoms at a younger age than non-carriers, but even for them that fate is not inevitable, and regular physical exercise may play an important role in an individual's outcome.

During these studies, the investigators performed PET scans that measured the amount of brain amyloid deposits in 201 people, ages 45 to 88. These amyloid protein deposits are associated with Alzheimer's disease symptoms. Volunteers with an active lifestyle had significantly less brain amyloid deposits compared with those with a sedentary lifestyle. The brain-healthy volunteers also had spinal fluid measures consistent with a healthier, amyloid-free brain. So regardless of your genetic predisposition, make an effort to exercise regularly—take a brisk walk, play tennis, swim, or do anything that gets your heart to pump oxygen and nutrients to your brain cells.

Q: **I read that scientists have discovered special immune proteins that attack Alzheimer's plaques in the brain. If those proteins are mass-produced, could that be a new cure?**

A: These special proteins are called monoclonal antibodies, and they stimulate an attack on the amyloid plaques associated with Alzheimer's disease. A recent study found that when the proteins were injected into patients with mild to moderate Alzheimer's dementia from two to seven times a month, the amount of their brain amyloid decreased by 15 percent compared with patients receiving placebo injections. Unfortunately, the patients receiving the proteins did not experience cognitive benefits. The treatment could have been too short to show a clinical effect, or these antibodies may only work in people at risk for dementia, before symptoms of Alzheimer's disease are obvious. To address this theory, prevention trials of these antibodies are currently in progress. Of course, it is also possible that clearing amyloid deposits from the brain is not effective in treating symptoms, and some other approach—fighting tau proteins or curtailing brain inflammation—is more effective.

Q: **Lots of people I know have started drinking coconut oil to protect them from Alzheimer's. Do you recommend it?**

A: Since Alzheimer's disease has no absolute cure, people are always pursuing new treatments, many based more on hope than actual science. In a recent book, a woman described how giving her husband 20 grams of coconut oil twice a day dramatically improved his Alzheimer's symptoms. Based on the idea that an Alzheimer's brain can't get enough glucose into its cells, providing another source of energy might help those cells get their nutrients and function better. Coconut oil contains fats that the liver converts to ketones, which the brain and other organs can use for energy.

The weakness of the coconut oil theory is that it is based on only one case. It is certainly worth further study, but many nutritionists are concerned about people consuming large amounts of coconut oil without any scientific basis since the oil contains saturated fats that can be harmful to heart health. Studies of laboratory animals fed saturated fats show that they develop high cholesterol levels, increases in brain amyloid, and impairment in memory abilities.

Q: **I'm becoming addicted to playing *Angry Birds* and other games on my cell phone. My wife says they're ridiculous and childish, but I say they exercise my brain. Who's right?**

A: Several studies suggest that playing action video games can improve some cognitive skills. Expert gamers are able to track moving objects at greater speeds and can switch mental tasks more rapidly than non-gamers. However, playing action video games has not been found to improve general cognitive skills involving memory and reasoning. Also, too much of something fun may not be good for you, especially if you have become addicted to the game. You might ask yourself what you are giving up when you spend so much time playing the game. Gaming addiction may draw you away from family, friends, work, and school, so both your personal and professional life might suffer. The key is to balance your *Angry Birds* time with low-tech activities that keep your life in balance, which will likely benefit your brain health most.

Q: **I was taking a lot of over-the-counter herbs and supplements to help my brain power, but my doctor said they don't work and they may be interacting with my blood-thinner medicine. What do you think?**

A: Your doctor is partially right. Some supplements do appear to improve brain function when they are tested against placebo. For example, phosphatidylserine, omega-3 fatty acids, vitamins D, $B_6$, and $B_{12}$, and folate have all been found to benefit cognitive abilities compared with placebo in studies lasting several months. However, long-term benefits have not been confirmed. Ginkgo biloba showed positive effects on memory in earlier studies, but the latest large-scale research has not confirmed these benefits. Also, ginkgo, as well as vitamin E, can increase the risk for bleeding especially if someone is taking Coumadin or a similar medicine that increases bleeding time.

Just like drug side effects, the potential adverse effects and drug interactions from herbal treatments are vast. The stimulating herb ginseng can cause headaches and anxiety. St. John's wort can help some people with depressive symptoms, but it can also interact with antidepressant drugs and some foods to cause side effects ranging from increased blood pressure to nausea and vomiting. You can check out websites (e.g., www.personalhealthzone.com/herbsafety .html) and other resources that provide details on these side effects and interactions; however, it's a good idea to tell your doctor about everything you're taking to ensure you don't run into problems.

## Q: I found a site on the Internet that asks a series of questions and then tells you whether you're getting Alzheimer's disease or not. Can I trust this site?

A: I would not trust any website that claims to be able to make a diagnosis of Alzheimer's disease by answering a series of questions online. A questionnaire can give a doctor information on the degree of memory challenges you are experiencing, but there are many causes of cognitive impairment, ranging from medication side effects to thyroid hormone imbalances. During the course of an evaluation for dementia or Alzheimer's, your doctor may ask a series of questions to determine the extent of cognitive impairment, but several other procedures are necessary. Your doctor needs to ask about your current symptoms and your past medical history. A thorough physical and neurological exam, as well as some laboratory tests, will help determine if a medical illness is contributing to symptoms. An MRI or CT scan is often performed to determine if a stroke or tumor is present, and a PET scan may show a pattern consistent with Alzheimer's disease.

## Q: I know that a good night's sleep improves my mental focus and energy level, but is there any direct link between sleep and risk for getting Alzheimer's?

A: Scientists at Washington University in St. Louis recently discovered that sleep patterns are related to Alzheimer's risk. Amyloid beta, the chemical that forms insoluble brain deposits in Alzheimer's disease, actually declines after about six hours of quality sleep.

# Additional Strategies for Working the Alzheimer's Prevention Program into Your Daily Routine

Some baby boomers who remain in the workforce are busy with their professional and personal lives and feel challenged to work the Alzheimer's Prevention Program into their daily routine. The following are suggestions on how to engage in a brain-healthy lifestyle while still completing the many tasks you have scheduled for your day.

- *Pick up the pace.* Walk briskly between destinations. A 10-minute errand can become a quick aerobic workout.
- *Divide the load.* If you are carrying heavy items, try to divide them evenly between hands to maintain balance. Of course, carrying a few pounds will offer some strength training for your arms. If possible, try doing a few bicep curls with the items while you continue your brisk walk.
- *Don't wait, meditate.* Those boring waits for a bus or elevator are opportunities to let go of frustration and relax—do some deep breathing, focus on releasing the tension from your neck and shoulder muscles. Pay attention to your posture (*stomach in, shoulders back*) or imagine yourself relaxing on a beach or in a hammock.
- *Schedule your exercises.* Set your smart phone to remind you to take a relaxation or brief exercise break every few hours. Stand up, stretch, and take a quick walk if you can. Try to get your heart pumping faster with some knee lifts or jumping jacks. If you've been at the computer for a couple of hours straight, interrupt your mental concentration by having a conversation with a friend or colleague or doing something different for a few minutes.
- *Jot it down.* To boost your brain power and minimize your tip-of-the-tongue memory slips, jot down some clues to the name or word that you think you should recall but can't. Look it up later and use *LOOK, SNAP, CONNECT* to sink it into your memory stores.

- *Carry a reminder or set your phone alarm.* Carry a wallet-sized card or set your phone alarm to remind you of the Alzheimer's Prevention Program exercises you are working on, whether it's *LOOK, SNAP, CONNECT,* names and faces, or a Sudoku puzzle.
- *Portion control.* Try splitting an entrée or a salad with a friend when dining at restaurants that serve oversized portions. If no one wants to share and you're trying to watch your weight, substitute an appetizer-sized dish for your entrée.
- *Surround yourself with healthy snacks.* Replace chocolates, donuts, and cookies with raisins, walnuts, and celery sticks. Keep a healthy energy bar (sugar should *not* be in the first three ingredients), not a candy bar, in your car, purse, or desk so you have it to snack on when you are feeling between-meal hunger pangs. Maintaining a steady stream of healthy nutrients to nourish your brain cells throughout the day is important to keeping them in optimal shape.

## Bonus Brain Teasers

1. WORD-FINDING FUN. Locate and circle all the words listed below, which can be found in the following diagram reading forward, backward, up, down, and diagonally, but always in a straight line. For extra credit, see how many additional words of three or more letters you can find after you locate all the listed words.

| | | | |
|---|---|---|---|
| AMYLOID | TAU | MEMORY | HIPPOCAMPUS |
| STRESS | CARDIO | BEET | VASCULAR |
| LOOK | SNAP | SOY | CONNECT |
| BRAIN | TEASER | NUT | DENDRITE |
| CARB | OLIVE | OIL | YAM |
| OMEGA | KICK | LIME | LIFT |
| CURRY | REM | VINE | RUN |

```
S   T   C   E   N   N   O   C   C   T   A
T   A   U   B   R   A   C   U   R   R   Y
R   A   L   U   C   S   A   V   I   N   E
E   S   O   Y   C   O   R   B   E   E   T
S   R   O   D   E   N   D   R   I   T   E
S   L   K   I   C   K   I   A   K   R   A
E   I   A   M   Y   L   O   I   D   N   S
R   F   O   M   E   G   A   N   O   N   E
T   T   R   E   M   M   S   S   A   O   R
S   U   P   M   A   C   O   P   P   I   H
S   N   Y   I   P   N   U   R   O   L   H
E   V   I   L   O   L   M   A   Y   P   O
```

2. **MENTAL MAGIC.** A memory expert throws a ball. The ball turns around 180 degrees mid-flight and returns to the memory expert. How did she do that?

3. **TRIVIA KNOWLEDGE.** Everyone knows that a bunch of cows is called a herd and that dogs bunch together in a pack, but what do you call a bunch of turtles?

4. **SCRAMBLED LETTERS.** See how many words of three letters or more you can write down, which include the letters below. (Each letter should be used only once in each word.) Set your timer for three minutes.

### S   L   M   E   O   I   P

___ ___ ___ ___ ___ ___ ___

5. **MOVING STICKS.** Take away six of the sticks below to make ten.

  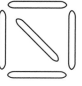

## ANSWERS TO BONUS BRAIN GAMES AND TEASERS

1. WORD-FINDING FUN. (Some of the answers are circled and others are shaded.)

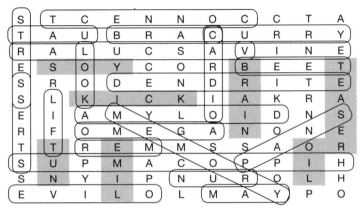

2. MENTAL MAGIC. She threw the ball straight up in the air.

3. TRIVIA KNOWLEDGE. A bunch of turtles is a bale.

4. SCRAMBLED LETTERS. Here are the words I wrote down. You may have found others as well:

ELM, ELMS
LEI, LIE, LIES, LIME, LIMES, LIP, LIPS, LOP, LOPS, LOPE, LOPES
MILE, MILES, MOP, MOPS, MOPE, MOPES
OLE, OPE, OPES
POEM, POEMS, POLE, POLES
SLIM, SLIME, SLOP, SLOPE

5. MOVING STICKS. Take away six of the sticks below to make ten.

 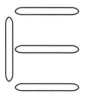

# Appendices

# Appendix 1: Progress Charts

The following blank charts can be helpful in plotting your progress for different exercises, as we did in Chapter 10. You can use graph paper to make similar kinds of charts if you find it helpful.

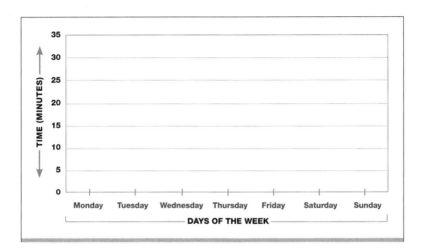

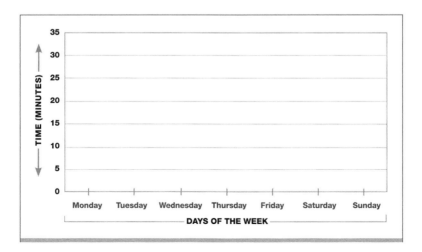

Here is another format that allows you to organize your activities and exercises.

| ACTIVITY | Monday | Tuesday | Wednesday | Thursday | Friday | Saturday | Sunday |
|---|---|---|---|---|---|---|---|
| | | | | | | | |
| | | | | | | | |
| | | | | | | | |
| | | | | | | | |
| | | | | | | | |
| | | | | | | | |
| | | | | | | | |
| | | | | | | | |
| | | | | | | | |
| | | | | | | | |
| | | | | | | | |
| | | | | | | | |

# Appendix 2: Additional Resources
# Educational and Advocacy Organizations

Many organizations provide information on general health and other topics that may help us improve cognitive abilities and brain health as we age. Several national organizations also have local or state chapters. Check your telephone directory or Internet search engine for related organizations and websites.

| NAME & ADDRESS | DESCRIPTION | TELEPHONE |
|---|---|---|
| **AARP**<br>6601 E St. N.W.<br>Washington, DC 20049<br>www.aarp.org | Nonprofit dedicated to helping older Americans live independently and with dignity and purpose. | 202-434-2277<br>800-424-3410 |
| **Administration on Aging**<br>330 Independence Ave. N.W.<br>Washington, DC 20201<br>www.aoa.gov | Provides information for older Americans and their families on opportunities and services to enrich their lives and support their independence. | 202-619-7501<br>800-677-1116 |
| **Aging Network Services**<br>4400 E. West Highway, Ste. 907<br>Bethesda, MD 20814<br>www.agingnets.com | Nationwide network of private-practice geriatric social workers serving as care managers for seniors. | 301-657-4329 |
| **Alzheimer Europe**<br>145 Route de Thionville<br>L-2611 Luxembourg<br>www.alzheimer-europe.org | Organizes caregiver support and raises awareness of dementia through cooperation among Alzheimer's organizations throughout Europe. | 352-29-7970 |
| **Alzheimer's Association**<br>919 N. Michigan Ave., Ste. 1000<br>Chicago, IL 60611<br>www.alz.org | National organization that provides information on services, programs, publications, and local chapters. | 800-272-3900 |
| **Alzheimer's Disease Education &**<br>**Referral Center**<br>P.O. Box 8250<br>Silver Spring, MD 20907<br>www.alzheimers.org | National Institute on Aging service that distributes information and free materials on topics relevant to health professionals, patients and their families, and the general public. | 301-495-3311<br>800-438-4380 |
| **Alzheimer's Foundation of**<br>**America**<br>322 Eighth Ave., 7th Flr.<br>New York, NY 10001<br>www.alzfdn.org | Nonprofit foundation supporting organizations that help lighten the burden and improve the quality of life of Alzheimer's patients and their caregivers. | 866-232-8484 |

|  |  |  |
|---|---|---|
| **American Academy of Neurology** 1080 Montreal Ave. St. Paul, MN 55116 www.aan.com | Professional organization that supports the art and science of neurology, thereby promoting the best possible care for patients with neurological disorders. | 651-695-1940 |
| **American Association for Geriatric Psychiatry** 7910 Woodmont Ave., Ste. 1050 Bethesda, MD 20814 www.aagpgpaonline.org | Professional organization dedicated to enhancing the mental health and well-being of older adults through education and research. | 301-654-7850 |
| **American Geriatrics Society** 770 Lexington Ave., Ste. 300 New York, NY 10021 www.americangeriatrics.org | Professional association that provides assistance with local geriatric physician referrals. | 212-308-1414 800-247-4779 |
| **American Psychiatric Association** 1000 Wilson Blvd., Ste. 1825 Arlington, VA 22209 www.psych.org | Medical specialty society that works to ensure humane care and effective treatment for all people with mental disorders. | 888-357-7924 |
| **American Psychological Association** 750 First St. N.E. Washington, DC 20002 www.apa.org | Scientific and professional organization that represents U.S. psychology and aims to promote health, education, and human welfare. | 800-374-2721 |
| **American Society on Aging** 833 Market St., Ste. 511 San Francisco, CA 94103 www.asaging.org | National organization concerned with physical, emotional, social, economic, and spiritual aspects of aging. | 415-974-9600 800-537-9728 |
| **www.clinicaltrials.gov** | Registry of federal and private clinical trials conducted in the U.S. and around the world, with information on contacts, locations, and trial purposes. | |
| **Dana Alliance for Brain Initiatives** 745 Fifth Ave., Ste. 900 New York, NY 10151 www.dana.org | Nonprofit organization committed to advancing public awareness of the progress and benefits of brain research. | 212-223-4040 |
| **Gerontological Society of America** 1030 15th St. N.W., Ste. 250 Washington, DC 20005 www.geron.org | National interdisciplinary organization on research and education in aging. | 202-842-1275 |
| **National Association of Area Agencies on Aging** 1730 Rhode Island Ave N.W., Ste. 1200 Washington, DC 20036 www.n4a.org | Umbrella organization for the local agencies on aging that help older people and people with disabilities live with dignity and choices in their homes and communities for as long as possible. | 202-872-0888 |

| | | |
|---|---|---|
| **National Center for Complementary and Alternative Medicine** P.O. Box 7923 Bethesda, MD 20898 www.nccam.nih.gov | The branch of the National Institutes of Health dedicated to exploring complementary and alternative healing practices in the context of rigorous science. | 888-644-6226 |
| **National Council on Aging** 409 Third St. S.W., Ste. 305 Washington, DC 20024 www.ncoa.org | A national network of organizations and individuals dedicated to improving the health and independence of older persons and increasing their continuing contributions to society. | 202-479-1200 |
| **National Institute of Mental Health** 5600 Fishers Ln., Rm. 10-75 Rockville, MD 20857 www.nimh.nih.gov | The branch of the National Institutes of Health that focuses on biomedical and behavioral research. | 301-443-1185 |
| **National Institute of Neurological Disorders and Stroke** NIH Neurological Institute P. O. Box 5801 Bethesda, MD 20824 www.ninds.nih.gov | The National Institutes of Health agency that supports neuroscience research; focuses on rapidly translating scientific discoveries into prevention, treatment, and cures; and provides resource support and information. | 301-496-5751 800-352-9424 |
| **National Institute on Aging** Bldg. 31, Rm. 5C27 31 Center Dr. MSC 2292 Bethesda, MD 20892-2292 www.nih.gov/nia | The National Institutes of Health agency that supports research on aging and provides information about national Alzheimer's centers and a free directory of organizations that serve older adults. | 301-496-1752 800-438-4380 |
| **National Stroke Association** 96 Inverness Dr. E., Ste. 1 Englewood, CO 80112-5112 www.stroke.org | Their mission is to reduce the incidence and impact of stroke and improve quality of patient care and outcomes. | 303-649-9299 800-787-6537 |
| **SeniorNet** 121 Second St., 7th Flr. San Francisco, CA 94105 www.seniornet.com | National nonprofit organization that works to build a community of computer-using seniors. | 415-495-4990 |
| **UCLA Longevity Center** 10945 Le Conte Ave., Ste. 3119 Los Angeles, CA 90095 www.longevity.ucla.edu | University center that works to enhance and extend productive and healthy life through research and education on aging. | 310-794-0676 |
| **U.S. Department of Veterans Affairs** 1120 Vermont Ave. N.W. Washington, DC 20421 www.va.gov | Provides information on veterans benefits, VA programs, VA facilities worldwide, and VA medical automation software. | 800-827-1000 |

# Brain Game Websites and Bonus Resources

Brain fitness is a burgeoning industry. Check out these and other websites to continue your mental stimulation program. Some of the sites offer free games, and others provide free samples before you sign up and pay for their programs and exercises. These games will increase your mental efficiency and can be a lot of fun.

www.brainbashers.com

www.brainden.com

www.brainteasers.org

www.luminosity.com

www.puzzle.dse.nl/index_us.html

www.sharpbrains.com

www.trickyriddles.com

## More Brain Game Online Resources

Dakim Brain Fitness:
www.dakim.com

Braingle: www.braingle.com

Posit Science:
www.positscience.com

Syvum: www.syvum.com/teasers

Pedagonet: www.pedagonet.com/
brain/brainers.html

Yahoo! Games:
http://games.yahoo.com

The Grey Labyrinth:
www.greylabyrinth.com

## Bonus Resources on Alzheimer's, Dementia, and Prevention

AARP on Brain Health:
www.aarp.org/health/
brain-health

Alzheimer's Association:
www.alz.org

Alzheimer's Foundation of America:
www.alzfdn.org

Alzheimer Research Forum:
www.alzforum.org

Alzheimer's Research UK:
www.alzheimersresearchuk.org

Alzheimer's Society:
alzheimers.org.uk

Fisher Center for Alzheimer's
Research Foundation:
www.alzinfo.org

Help Guide: http://helpguide.org/
elder/alzheimers_prevention_
slowing_down_treatment.htm

# Appendix 3: Notes and Scientific References

## CHAPTER 1

*Large-scale surveys show that more than:* Alzheimer's Foundation of America survey. www .alzfdn.org/MediaCenter/073008.html.

Ginó, S., et al. "Memory complaints are frequent but qualitatively different in young and elderly healthy people." *Gerontology* 56 (2010): 272–77.

*Baby boomers are quite aware of the rising tide:* Alzheimer's Association. *2009 Alzheimer's Disease Facts and Figures.* www.alz.org/national/documents/report_alzfactsfigures2009 .pdf.

*In 2010 the estimated worldwide costs:* Alzheimer's Disease International. *World Alzheimer's Report 2010: The Global Economic Impact of Dementia.* www.alz.org/documents/ national/World_Alzheimer_Report_2010.pdf.

*Science has shown that genetics:* Rowe, J. W., and R. L. Kahn. "The future of aging." *Contemp Longterm Care* 22 (1999): 36–44.

*In 1906 Alois Alzheimer presented:* Graeber, M. B., et al. "Histopathology and APOE genotype of the first Alzheimer disease patient, Auguste D." *Neurogenetics* 1 (1998): 223–28.

*In the late 1960s, however, neuropathologists:* Blessed, G., et al. "The association between quantitative measures of dementia and of senile change in the cerebral grey matter of elderly subjects." *Br J Psychiatry* 114 (1968): 797–811.

*A recent NIH consensus panel:* Daviglus, M. L., et al. NIH State-of-the-Science Conference Statement on Preventing Alzheimer's Disease and Cognitive Decline. *NIH Consens State Sci Statements* 27 (2010): 1–30.

*When neuropathologists looked at hundreds:* Braak, H., and E. Braak. "Neuropathological staging of Alzheimer-related changes." *Acta Neuropathol* 82 (1991): 239–59.

*But in 2002, our UCLA research team discovered:* Shoghi-Jadid, K., et al. "Localization of neurofibrillary tangles and beta-amyloid plaques in the brains of living patients with Alzheimer's disease." *Am J Geriatr Psychiatry* 10 (2002): 24–35.

*Since this initial discovery, we have studied hundreds of people:* Small, G. W., et al. "PET of brain amyloid and tau in mild cognitive impairment." *N Engl J Med* 355 (2006): 2652–63.

Small, G. W., et al. "Influence of cognitive status, age, and APOE-4 genetic risk on brain FDDNP positron-emission tomography imaging in persons without dementia." *Arch Gen Psychiatry* 66 (2009): 81–87.

Ercoli, L. M., et al. "Differential FDDNP PET patterns in non-demented middle-aged and older adults." *Am J Geriatr Psychiatry* 17 (2009): 397–406.

*. . . I prescribed Aricept:* Petersen, R. C., et al. "Vitamin E and donepezil for the treatment of mild cognitive impairment." *N Engl J Med* 352 (2005): 2379–88.

*Dr. Ron Petersen of the Mayo Clinic:* Petersen, R. C. "Mild cognitive impairment as a diagnostic entity." *J Int Med* 256 (2004): 183–94.

*Experts have revised the definitions for:* Dubois, B., et al. "Revising the definition of Alzheimer's disease: A new lexicon." *Lancet Neurol* 9 (2010): 1118–27.

"New Criteria and Guidelines for Alzheimer's Disease Diagnosis." *Alzheim Dementia* 2011. www.alzheimersanddementia.org/content/ncg.

*Mme. Jeanne Calment of France was free of Alzheimer's disease:* Ritchie, K. "Eugeria, longevity and normal ageing." *Br J Psychiatry* 171 (1997): 501.

*I participated in a national consensus:* Relkin, N. R., et al. "Apolipoprotein E genotyping in Alzheimer's disease: Position statement of the National Institute on Aging/Alzheimer's Association Working Group." *Lancet* 347 (1996): 1091–95.

*Years later, Dr. Robert Green:* Ashida, S., et al. "The role of disease perceptions and results sharing in psychological adaptation after genetic susceptibility testing: the REVEAL Study." *Eur J Hum Genet* 18 (2010): 1296–1301.

*The MacArthur Study of Successful Aging taught:* Rowe, J. W., and R. L. Kahn. "The future of aging." *Contemp Longterm Care* 22 (1999): 36–44.

*our UCLA group studied several sets of identical twins:* Small G. W., et al. "Clinical, neuroimaging, and environmental risk differences in monozygotic female twins appearing discordant for dementia of the Alzheimer type." *Arch Neurol* 50 (1993): 209–19.

*some of the latest studies of antiplaque treatments have failed:* Smith, A. D. "Why are drug trials in Alzheimer's disease failing?" *Lancet* 376 (2010): 1466.

Extance, A. "Alzheimer's failure raises questions about disease-modifying strategies." *Nat Rev Drug Discov* 9 (2010): 749–51.

*researchers have discovered tiny proteins, called oligomers:* Tomic, J. L., et al. "Soluble fibrillar oligomer levels are elevated in Alzheimer's disease brain and correlate with cognitive dysfunction." *Neurobiol Dis* 35 (2009): 352–58.

*the results of the Baltimore Longitudinal Study:* Stewart, W. F., et al. "Risk of Alzheimer's disease and duration of NSAID use." *Neurology* 48 (1997): 626–32.

*my UCLA research team conducted a double-blind study:* Small, G. W., et al. "Cognitive and cerebral metabolic effects of celecoxib versus placebo in people with age-related memory loss: Randomized controlled study." *Am J Geriatr Psychiatry* 16 (2008): 999–1009.

*Dr. John Breitner and his coworkers:* Sonnen, J. A., et al. "Nonsteroidal anti-inflammatory drugs are associated with increased neuritic plaques." *Neurology* 75 (2010): 1203–10.

Breitner, J.C.S. and P. P. Zandi. "Do nonsteroidal anti-inflammatory drugs reduce the risk of Alzheimer's disease?" *N Engl J Med* 345 (2001): 1567–78.

*Considerable scientific evidence points to lifestyle:* Jerdziewski, M. K., et al. "Lowering the risk of Alzheimer's disease: Evidence-based practices emerge from new research." *Alzheimer Dement* 1 (2005): 152–60.

Rolland, Y., et al. "Healthy brain aging: Role of exercise and physical activity." *Clin Geriatr Med* 26 (2010): 75–87.

Sofi, F., et al. "Effectiveness of the Mediterranean diet: Can it help delay or prevent Alzheimer's disease?" *J Alzheim Dis* 20 (2010): 795–801.

Lee, Y., et al. "Systematic review of health behavioral risks and cognitive health in older adults." *Int Psychogeriatr* 22 (2010): 174–87.

Desai, A. K., et al. "Healthy brain aging: A road map." *Clin Geriatr Med* 25 (2010): 1–16.

*Although some experts have called for additional long-term studies:* Daviglus, M. L., et al. "NIH State-of-the-Science Conference Statement on Preventing Alzheimer's Disease and Cognitive Decline." *NIH Consens State Sci Statements* 27 (2010): 1–30.

Daviglus, M. L., B. L. Plassman, A. Pirzada, et al. "Risk factors and preventive interventions for Alzheimer disease: State of the science." *Arch Neurol* 100 (2011): 1–6.

*In our UCLA collaboration with the RAND Corporation:* Woo, S. Y., and G. W. Small. "Aging Forecast." UCLA Center on Aging (2003).

*In fact, an estimated six million people:* Alzheimer's Association. *Changing the Trajectory of Alzheimer's disease: A National Imperative.* www.alz.org/documents_custom/trajectory.pdf.

*We can estimate the potential impact of a healthy lifestyle:* Etgen, T., et al. "Physical activity and incident cognitive impairment in elderly persons: The INVADE study." *Arch Intern Med* 170 (2010): 186–93.

Morris, M. C., et al. "Relation of the tocopherol forms to incident Alzheimer disease and to cognitive change." *Am J Clin Nutr* 81 (2005): 508–14.

Karp, A., et al. "Mentally stimulating activities at work during midlife and dementia risk after age 75: Follow-up study from the Kungsholmen Project." *Am J Geriatr Psychiatry* 17 (2009): 227–36.

*if Jack continued his walks for four years:* This estimate is based on the calculation of a 1.8-year delay, assuming a 46 percent risk reduction over two years from the epidemiological studies.

*then Jack's Alzheimer's symptoms could be staved off:* If we factor in Jack's exercising (46 percent protective effect in lowering dementia risk over two years, equivalent to 23 percent per year) and healthy eating (44 percent protective effect over four years, equivalent to an additional 11 percent per year), then the new estimated protective effect based on the epidemiological studies would be the sum of the effects of the two new habits..

*Systematic studies have documented these positive outcomes:* Small, G. W., et al. "Effects of a 14-day healthy longevity lifestyle program on cognition and brain function." *Am J Geriatr Psychiatry* 14 (2006): 538–45.

Miller, K. J., et al. "The Memory Fitness Program: Cognitive effects of a healthy aging intervention." *Am J Geriatr Psychiatry* 20 (2012): 514–23.

*Other studies have reported similar kinds of synergy:* Knowler, W. C., et al: "Reduction in the incidence of type 2 diabetes with lifestyle intervention or metformin. *N Engl J Med* 346 (2002): 393–403.

Blumenthal, J. A., et al: "Usefulness of psychosocial treatment of mental stress-induced myocardial ischemia in men." *Am J Cardiol* 89 (2002): 164–68.

Eapen, D. J., et al. "Raising HDL cholesterol in women." *Int J Women Health* 1 (2010): 181–91.

## CHAPTER 2

*Systematic studies have confirmed that this type of knowledge:* Sarkisian, C. A., et al. "Pilot test of an attribution retraining intervention to raise walking levels in sedentary older adults." *J Am Geriatr Soc* 55 (2007): 1842–46.

*The questionnaires and assessment scales are adapted from those I have used:* Small, G. W., et al. "Mnemonics usage and cognitive decline in age-associated memory impairment." *Int Psychogeriatr* 9 (1997): 47–56.

Ercoli, L. M., et al. "Perceived loss of memory ability and cerebral metabolic decline in persons with the apolipoprotein E-4 genetic risk for Alzheimer's disease." *Arch Gen Psychiatry* 63 (2006): 442–48.

*Our UCLA brain scan studies have shown that memory self-assessment:* Small, G. W., et al. "Memory self-appraisal and depressive symptoms in people at genetic risk for Alzheimer's disease." *Int J Geriatr Psychiatry* 16 (2001): 1071–77.

Merrill, D. A., et al. "Memory self-appraisal and PET of brain amyloid and tau in persons without dementia." *Abstracts from the 15th Annual UCLA Research Conference on Aging* (2010).

*aerobic training improves brain function as we age:* Voss, M. V., et al. "Plasticity of brain networks in a randomized intervention trial of exercise training in older adults." *Front Aging Neurosci* 2 (2010): 32.

*The National Institutes of Health have provided a formula:* "Weight Management," www .nlm.nih.gov/medlineplus/ency/article/001943.htm.

*Chronic stress not only diminishes our quality of life:* Wilson, R. S., et al. "Proneness to psychological distress is associated with risk of Alzheimer's disease." *Neurology* 61 (2003): 1479–85.

## CHAPTER 3

*Neuroscientists at Yale University found that when the brain is cluttered:* Kuhl, B. A., et al. "Fidelity of neural reactivation reveals competition between memories." *Proc Natl Acad Sci USA* 108 (2011): 5903–08.

*UCLA scientists have found significantly higher quantities of white matter:* Bartzokis, G., et al. "Lifespan trajectory of myelin integrity and maximum motor speed." *Neurobiol Aging* 31 (2010): 1554–62.

*improved mental abilities when both sides of the brain work on a task together:* Cabeza, R., et al. "Aging gracefully: Compensatory brain activity in high-performing older adults." *NeuroImage* 17 (2002): 1394–1402.

*In people with mild cognitive impairment, memory training not only improves:* Belleville, S., et al. "Training-related brain plasticity in subjects at risk of developing Alzheimer's disease." *Brain* 134 (2011): 1623–34.

*My UCLA research indicates that the memory abilities of people who have a genetic risk:* Bookheimer, S. Y., et al. "Patterns of brain activation in people at risk for Alzheimer's disease." *N Engl J Med* 343 (2000): 450–56.

*Scientific evidence shows that practicing simple memory techniques:* Buschert, V., et al. "Cognitive intervention in Alzheimer disease." *Nature* 6 (2010): 508–17.

*Our UCLA research group has found that using basic memory methods can activate:* Small, G. W., et al. "Your brain on Google: Patterns of cerebral activation during Internet searching." *Am J Geriatr Psychiatry* 17 (2009): 116–26.

Small, G. W., et al. "Effects of a 14-day healthy longevity lifestyle program on cognition and brain function." *Am J Geriatr Psychiatry* 14 (2006): 538–45.

*For example, a ten-session memory training course:* Willis, S. L., et al. "Long-term effects of cognitive training on everyday functional outcomes in older adults." *JAMA* 296 (2006): 2805–14.

*In 2010, Wang Feng won the World Memory Championships:* World Memory Championships website: www.worldmemorychampionships.com.

## CHAPTER 4

*the fitness habits of 18-year-olds predicted their educational achievements later in life:* Aberg, M.A.I., et al. "Cardiovascular fitness is associated with cognition in young adulthood." *Proc Natl Acad Sci USA* 106 (2009): 20, 906–11.

*A 2010 report from the Framingham Longitudinal Study:* Tan, Z. S., et al. "Physical activity and the risk of dementia: The Framingham Study." International Conference on Alzheimer's Disease, July 2010.

*In a study of more than 18,000 older women:* Weuve, J., et al. "Physical activity, including walking, and cognitive function in older women." *JAMA* 292 (2004): 1454–61.

*University of Pittsburgh scientists found that the more:* Raji, C., et al. "Physical activity and gray matter volume in late adulthood: The Cardiovascular Health Cognition Study." Radiological Society of North America, 28 Nov 2010; SSA17-01.

*Dr. Arthur Kramer and colleagues:* Colcombe, S. J., et al. "Cardiovascular fitness, cortical plasticity, and aging." *Proc Natl Acad Sci USA* 101 (2004): 3316–21.

Voss, M. W., et al. "Plasticity of brain networks in a randomized intervention trial of exercise training in older adults." *Front Aging Neurosci* 2 (2010): 1–17.

*Other research indicates that just 20 minutes of daily aerobic exercise can improve memory:* Lautenschlager, N. T., et al. "Effect of physical activity on cognitive function in older adults at risk for Alzheimer disease." *JAMA* 300 (2008): 1027–37.

*In one recent investigation, Brazilian:* Cassilhas, R. C., et al. "The impact of 8 weeks of aerobic or resistance exercise on spatial memory and hippocampal BDNF of rodents." *Annual Meeting of the Society for Neuroscience* 2010: 635.1.

*Japanese researchers increased the resistance of the running wheels:* Minchul, L., et al. "Loaded wheel running enhance BDNF function in the rat hippocampus." *Annual Meeting of the Society for Neuroscience* 2010: 337.11/E18.

*Dr. Teresa Liu-Ambrose found that weight lifters have better cognitive abilities:* Liu-Ambrose, T., et al. "Resistance training and executive functions: A 12-month randomized controlled trial." *Arch Intern Med* 170 (2010): 170–78.

*Our UCLA studies have found that some symptoms of depression:* Lavretsky, H., et al. "Depression and anxiety symptoms are associated with cerebral FDDNP-PET binding in middle-aged and older adults." *Am J Geriatr Psychiatry* 17 (2009): 493–502.

*Colleagues from Duke University recently compared the antidepressant effects of aerobic exercise:* Blumenthal, J. A., et al. "Exercise and pharmacotherapy in the treatment of major depressive disorder." *Psychosom Med* 69 (2007): 587–96.

*Research from economist George Loewenstein at Carnegie Mellon University:* Rick, S., et al. "Tightwads and spendthrifts." *J Consumer Res* 34 (2008): 767–82.

*Systematic studies have found that multiple periods of brief exercise:* Schmidt, W. D., et al. "Effects of long versus short bout exercise on fitness and weight loss in overweight females." *J Am Coll Nutrition* 20 (2001): 494–501.

*Brain scans of experienced dancers show strengthened neural circuits:* Pilgramm, S., et al. "Differential activation of the lateral premotor cortex during action observation." *BMC Neurosci* 11 (2010): 89.

*Ruhr-University scientists in Germany:* Kattenstroth, J. C., et al. "Superior sensory, motor, and cognitive performance in elderly individuals with multi-year dancing activities." *Front Aging Neurosci* 2 (21 Jul 2010) pii: 31.

*Investigators at the University of Missouri College of Veterinary Medicine:* Johnson, R. A., and R. L. Meadows. "Dog-walking: motivation for adherence to a walking program." *Clin Nurs Res* 19 (2010): 387–402.

*Most people think of weight lifting as a sport reserved for young:* Latham, N., and C. J. Liu.

Strength training in older adults: the benefits for osteoarthritis." *Clin Geriatr Med* 26 (2010): 445–59.

*Older research volunteers who incorporate balance training:* Williamson, J. D., et al. "Changes in cognitive function in a randomized trial of physical activity: Results of the lifestyle interventions and independence for elders pilot study." *J Gerontol A Biol Sci Med Sci* 64 (2009): 688–94.

*Investigators at Aristotle University of Thessaloniki, in Greece:* Sofianidis, G., et al. "Effect of a 10-week traditional dance program on static and dynamic balance control in elderly adults." *J Aging Phys Act* 17 (2009): 167–80.

*Other studies have found that older adults who are regular social dancers:* Verghese, J. "Cognitive and mobility profile of older social dancers." *J Am Geriatr Soc* 54 (2006): 1241–44.

*A recent study found that middle-aged people who attended a 12-week Pilates class:* Kloubec, J. A. "Pilates for improvement of muscle endurance, flexibility, balance, and posture." *J Strength Cond Res* 24 (2010): 661–67.

*Researchers at Bond University, in Australia:* Sekendiz, B., et al. "Effects of swiss-ball core strength training on strength, endurance, flexibility, and balance in sedentary women." *J Strength Cond Res* 24 (2010): 3032–40.

## CHAPTER 5

*A recent Columbia University study:* Gu, Y., et al. "Food combination and Alzheimer disease risk: A protective diet." *Arch Neurol* 67 (2010): 699–706.

*Today, nearly 73 million Americans are obese:* Centers for Disease Control and Prevention. *Overweight and Obesity: U.S. Obesity Trends.* www.cdc.gov/obesity/data/trends.html.

*It also impairs brain health:* Hassing, L. B., et al. "Overweight in midlife and risk of dementia: A 40-year follow-up study." *Int J Obes (Lond)* 33 (2009): 893–98.

*In a four-year study of more than 7,000 French volunteers:* Raffaitin, C., et al. "Metabolic syndrome and risk for incident Alzheimer's disease or vascular dementia: The Three-City Study." *Diabetes Care* 32 (2009): 169–74.

*In a study of more than 2,000 healthy individuals:* Cournot, M., et al. "Relation between body mass index and cognitive function in healthy middle-aged men and women." *Neurology* 67 (2006): 1208–14.

*Researchers from Boston University School of Medicine:* Debette, S., et al. "Visceral fat is associated with lower brain volume in healthy middle-aged adults." *Ann Neurol* 68 (2010): 136–44.

*Neuroscientists have found evidence that as BMI rises:* Gazdzinski, S., et al. "BMI and neuronal integrity in healthy, cognitively normal elderly: A proton magnetic resonance spectroscopy study. *Obesity* 18 (2010): 743–48.

*A 2010 study published in* Science *magazine:* Morewedge, C. K., et al. "Thought for food: Imagined consumption reduces actual consumption." *Science* 330 (2010): 1530–33.

*Researchers at the University of Bristol, in the UK, found,:* Oldham, R. E., et al. "Playing a computer game during lunch affects fullness, memory for lunch, and later snack intake." *Am J Clin Nutr* 93 (2011): 308–13.

*Researchers have now pinpointed a network of brain regions associated:* Wang, G. J., et al. "Gastric distention activates satiety circuitry in the human brain." *NeuroImage* 39 (2008): 1824–31.

*Some studies have found that very low carbohydrate diets:* Brehm, B. J., et al. "A randomized trial comparing a very low carbohydrate diet and a calorie-restricted low fat diet on body weight and cardiovascular risk factors in healthy women." *J Clin Endocrinol Metab* 88 (2003): 1617–23.

*Being overweight throws off our immune systems:* Zhou, Q., et al. "Signaling mechanisms in the restoration of impaired immune function due to diet-induced obesity." *Proc Natl Acad Sci USA* 108 (2011): 2867–72.

*a low-calorie diet can alter the expression of inflammatory genes:* Mraz, M., et al. "The effect of very-low-calorie diet on mRNA expression of inflammation-related genes in subcutaneous adipose tissue and peripheral monocytes of obese patients with type 2 diabetes mellitus." *J Clin Endocrinol Metab* 96 (2011): E606–13.

*Spices and aromatic herbs also have anti-inflammatory effects:* Viuda-Martos, M., et al. Spices as functional foods. *Crit Rev Food Sci Nutr* 51 (2011): 13–28.

*compounds known as flavonoids:* Xiao, Z. P., et al. "Flavonoids health benefits and their molecular mechanism." *Mini Rev Med Chem* 11 (2011): 169–77.

*but the amount of turkey one would need to ingest in order to have a mental effect:* Greenwood, M. H., et al. "The acute effects of oral (--)-tryptophan in human subjects." *Br J Clin Pharmacol* 2 (1975): 165–72.

Holden J., Nutrient Data Laboratory, USDA, Agricultural Research Service. "USDA National Nutrient Database for Standard Reference, Release 22." United States Department of Agriculture. www.ars.usda.gov/ba/bhnrc/ndl.

*Multiple studies have shown that omega-3s have an antidepressant effect:* Rocha Araujo, D. M., et al. "What is the effectiveness of the use of polyunsaturated fatty acid omega-3 in the treatment of depression?" *Expert Rev Neurother* 10 (2010): 1117–29.

*The Rotterdam Study:* Rocha Araujo, D. M., et al. "Dietary antioxidants and long-term risk of dementia." *Arch Neurol* 67 (2010): 819–25.

*In another large-scale European study, of more than 8,000:* Barberger-Gateau, P., et al. "Dietary patterns and risk of dementia: The Three-City cohort study." *Neurology* 69 (2007): 1921–30.

*Low levels of antioxidants in the blood:* Goyarzu, P., et al. "Blueberry supplemented diet: Effects on object recognition memory and nuclear factor-kappa B levels in aged rats." *Nutr Neurosci* 7 (2004): 75–83.

*The tables on page 97 . . . list examples of some fruits and vegetables:* USDA, Agricultural Research Service. "Oxygen Radical Absorbance Capacity (ORAC) of Selected Foods, Release 2." May 2010. www.ars.usda.gov/Services/docs.htm?docid=15866.

*Investigators from Vanderbilt School of Medicine:* Dai, Q., et al. "Fruit and vegetable juices and Alzheimer's disease: The Kame Project." *Am J Med* 119 (2006): 751–59.

*Experimental Alzheimer's mice that drank pomegranate juice:* Hartman, R. E., et al. "Pomegranate juice decreases amyloid load and improves behavior in a mouse model of Alzheimer's disease." *Neurobiol Dis* 24 (2006): 506–15.

*green tea is another good source of antioxidants:* Kim, J., et al. "Naturally occurring phytochemicals for the prevention of Alzheimer's disease." *J Neurochem* 112 (2010): 1415–30.

*people who consume large amounts of these anti-inflammatory omega-3 fatty acids:* Cole, G. M., et al. "Omega-3 fatty acids and dementia." *Prostaglandins Leukot Essent Fatty Acids* 81 (2009): 213–21.

*Studies comparing rates of dementia in Nigerians:* Ogunniyi, A., et al. "Epidemiology of dementia in Nigeria: Results from the Indianapolis-Ibadan study." *Eur J Neurol* 7 (2000): 485–90.

*One study of restaurant goers:* Wansink, B., and L. R. Linder. "Interactions between forms of fat consumption and restaurant bread consumption." *Int J Obes Relat Metab Disord* 27 (2003): 866–68.

*In their study of food combinations:* Gu, Y., et al. "Food combination and Alzheimer disease risk: A protective diet." *Arch Neurol* 67 (2010): 699–706.

*Research suggests that a low GI diet may decrease the risk for developing diabetes:* Sluijs, I., et al. "Carbohydrate quantity and quality and risk of type 2 diabetes in the European Prospective Investigation into Cancer and Nutrition–Netherlands (EPIC-NL) study." *Am J Clin Nutr* 92 (2010): 905–11.

*Investigators from the Cooper Institute in Dallas, Texas:* Finley, C. E., et al. "Glycemic index, glycemic load, and prevalence of the metabolic syndrome in the Cooper center longitudinal study." *J Am Diet Assoc* 110 (2010): 1820–29.

*A recent study that included nearly 15,000 participants:* Anstey, K. J., et al. "Alcohol consumption as a risk factor for dementia and cognitive decline: Meta-analysis of prospective studies." *Am J Geriatr Psychiatry* 17 (2009): 542–55.

*Scientists at Mount Sinai School of Medicine, in New York, studied the effects of wine:* Wang, J., et al. "Moderate consumption of Cabernet Sauvignon attenuates Abeta neuropathology in a mouse model of Alzheimer's disease." *FASEB J* 20 (2006): 2313–20.

*A large-scale epidemiological study from Sweden reported that drinking:* Eskelinen, M. H., and M. Kivipelto. "Caffeine as a protective factor in dementia and Alzheimer's disease." *J Alzheim Dis* 20, Suppl 1 (2010): S167–74.

*University of North Carolina scientists reported:* Chen, X., et al. "Caffeine protects against disruptions of the blood-brain barrier in animal models of Alzheimer's and Parkinson's diseases." *J Alzheim Dis* 20m Suppl 1 (2010): S127–41.

*For example, consuming garlic lowers:* Tapsell, L. C., et al. "Health benefits of herbs and spices: The past, the present, the future." *Med J Aust* 185 (2006): S4–24.

*The table on page 106 illustrates the strong antioxidant potencies:* Adapted from USDA, Agricultural Research Service. "Oxygen Radical Absorbance Capacity (ORAC) of Selected Foods, Release 2." May 2010. www.ars.usda.gov/Services/docs.htm?docid=15866. ORAC units in the table were adjusted to amounts corresponding to ½ ounce of each spice rather than the 3½ ounces indicated in the original experiment.

*Scientists recently studied piperine:* Chonpathompikunlert, P., et al. "Piperine, the main alkaloid of Thai black pepper, protects against neurodegeneration and cognitive impairment in animal model of cognitive deficit like condition of Alzheimer's disease." *Food Chem Toxicol* 48 (2010): 798–802.

*because of relatively lower rates of dementia in India:* Banerjee, T. K., et al. "Cognitive dysfunction in an urban Indian population—some observations." *Neuroepidemiology* 31 (2008): 109–14.

*My UCLA colleagues Drs. Greg Cole and Sally Frautschy:* Cole, G. M., et al. "Neuroprotective effects of curcumin." *Adv Exp Med Biol* 595 (2007): 197–212.

*In one study of more than 1,000 volunteers:* Ng, T. P., et al. "Curry consumption and cognitive function in the elderly." *Am J Epidemiol* 164 (2006): 898–906.

*The scientific evidence is compelling:* Gomez-Pinilla, F. "Brain foods: The effects of nutrients on brain function." *Nature Reviews* 9 (2008): 568–78.

## CHAPTER 6

*multiple studies reporting a connection between stimulating mental activities:* Hall, C. B., et al. "Cognitive activities delay onset of memory decline in persons who develop dementia." *Neurology* 73 (2009): 356–61.

Akbaraly, T. N., et al. "Leisure activities and the risk of dementia in the elderly: Results from the Three-City Study." *Neurology* 73 (2009): 854–61.

Lachman, M. E., et al. "Frequent cognitive activity compensates for education differences in episodic memory." *Am J Geriatr Psychiatry* 18 (2010): 4–10.

*Dr. Fred Gage and colleagues . . . reported that primitive neural stem cells:* Eriksson, P. S., et al. "Neurogenesis in the adult human hippocampus." *Nat Med* 4 (1998): 1313–17.

*People who inherit a healthy form of BDNF:* Voineskos, A. N., et al. "The brain-derived neurotrophic factor val66met polymorphism and prediction of neural risk for Alzheimer disease." *Arch Gen Psychiatry* 68 (2011): 198–206.

*higher BDNF blood levels are associated with exercise-induced enlargement:* Erickson, K. I., et al. "Exercise training increases size of hippocampus and improves memory." *Proc Natl Acad Sci USA* 108 (2011): 3017–22.

*Functional MRI studies also show that BDNF gene expression influences neural activity:* Hariri, A. R., et al. "Brain-derived neurotrophic factor val66met polymorphism affects human memory-related hippocampal activity and predicts memory performance." *J Neurosci* 23 (2003): 6690–94.

*After just seven hours of Internet:* Moody, T. D., et al. "Neural activity patterns in older adults following Internet training." Society for Neuroscience, 2009.

*Other experiments have shown that the brain recruits fewer neurons:* Small, G. W., et al. "Effects of a 14-day healthy longevity lifestyle program on cognition and brain function." *Am J Geriatr Psychiatry* 14 (2006): 538–45.

Haier, R. J., et al: "Regional glucose metabolic changes after learning a complex visuospatial/motor task: A positron emission tomographic study." *Brain Res* 570 (1992): 134–43.

*Recent research has confirmed earlier studies showing a connection between mental stimulation:* Hall, C. B., et al. "Cognitive activities delay onset of memory decline in persons who develop dementia." *Neurology* 73 (2009): 356–61.

Akbaraly, T. N., et al. "Leisure activities and the risk of dementia in the elderly: Results from the Three-City Study." *Neurology* 73 (2009): 854–61.

*Animal studies provide additional evidence that mental stimulation improves:* Gage, F. H. "Neurogenesis in the adult brain." *J Neurosci* 22 (2002): 612–13.

*Dr. Margie Lachman and colleagues at Brandeis University confirmed earlier:* Lachman, M. E., et al. "Frequent cognitive activity compensates for education differences in episodic memory." *Am J Geriatr Psychiatry* 18 (2010): 4–10.

*At UCLA our research team was able:* Moody, T. D., et al. "Neural activity patterns in older adults following Internet training." Society for Neuroscience, 2009.

*When psychologists provide specific training to improve short-term, or working, memory:* Jaeggi, S. M., et al. "Improving fluid intelligence with training on working memory." *Proc Natl Acad Sci USA* 105 (2008): 6829–33.

*Neuroscientists have found that during midlife our neurons may be especially agile:* Bartzokis, G., et al. "Apolipoprotein E genotype and age-related myelin breakdown in healthy individuals: Implications for cognitive decline and dementia." *Arch Gen Psychiatry* 63 (2006): 63–72.

*Another advantage to an older brain is that both sides:* Cabeza, R., et al. "Aging gracefully: Compensatory brain activity in high-performing older adults." *NeuroImage* 17 (2002): 1394–402.

*social interactions boost cognitive ability:* Ybarra, O., et al. "Mental exercising through simple socializing: Social interaction promotes general cognitive functioning." *Pers Soc Psychol Bull* 34 (2008): 248–59.

*Interacting with other people also helps us:* Wilson, R. S., et al. "Loneliness and risk of Alzheimer disease." *Arch Gen Psychiatry* 64 (2007): 234–40.

*Dr. Steven Cole and associates:* Cole, S. W., et al. "Transcript origin analysis identifies antigen-presenting cells as primary targets of socially regulated gene expression in leukocytes." *Proc Natl Acad Sci USA* 108 (2011): 3080–85.

*staying socially engaged may reduce your risk for dementia:* Wang, H.-X., et al. "Late-life engagement in social and leisure activities is associated with a decreased risk of dementia: A longitudinal study from the Kungsholmen Project." *Am J Epidemiol* 155 (2002): 1081–87.

*Unfamiliar stimuli and new mental challenges stimulate neuronal growth:* Hobson, J. A., and A. B. Scheibel. "The brainstem core: Sensorimotor integration and behavioral state control." *Neurosci Res Program Bull* 18 (1980): 1–173.

*Psychologist Ellen Bialystok and associates in Toronto, Canada, found that people who speak:* Craik, F. I., et al. "Delaying the onset of Alzheimer disease: Bilingualism as a form of cognitive reserve." *Neurology* 75 (2010): 1726–29.

*Brain scan studies show that we can build brain muscle specific:* Maguire, E. A., et al. "Navigation around London by a taxi driver with bilateral hippocampal lesions." *Brain* 129 (2006): 2894–907.

Boyke, J., et al. "Training-induced brain structure changes in the elderly." *J Neurosci* 28 (2008): 7031–35.

Matsumoto, R. et al. "Left anterior temporal cortex actively engages in speech perception: A direct cortical stimulation study." *Neuropsychologia* 49 (2011): 1350–54.

*Some experts estimate that by 2015:* Hafner, K.. "Exercise your brain, or else you'll . . . Uh . . ." *New York Times*, May 2, 2008: www.nytimes.com/2008/05/03/technology/03brain.html.

*The debate was recently fueled by a study published in the journal* Nature: Owen, A. M., et al. "Putting brain training to the test." *Nature* 465 (2010): 775–78.

*people who delay retirement by several years have better cognitive abilities:* Roberts, B. A., et al. "Does retirement influence cognitive performance? The Whitehall II Study." *J Epidemiol Community Health* doi:10.1136/jech.2010.111849.

## CHAPTER 7

*Dr. Lena Johansson and colleagues at the University of Gothenburg, in Sweden:* Johansson, L., et al. "Midlife psychological stress and risk of dementia: A 35-year longitudinal population study." *Brain* 133 (2010): 2217–24.

*Investigators at Rush University Medical Center, in Chicago:* Wilson, R. S., et al. "Proneness to psychological distress is associated with risk of Alzheimer's disease." *Neurology* 61 (2003): 1479–85.

Wilson, R. S., et al. "Chronic psychological distress and risk of Alzheimer's disease in old age." *Neuroepidemiology* 27 (2006): 143–53.

*Many studies have shown that older people with symptoms of depression:* Palmer, K., et al. "Predictors of progression from mild cognitive impairment to Alzheimer disease." *Neurology* 68 (2007): 1596–602.

Jorm, A. F. "Is depression a risk factor for dementia or cognitive decline? A review." *Gerontology* 46 (2000): 219–27.

*Depression has immediate effects on mental capacity:* Vitaliano, P. P., et al. "Depressed mood mediates decline in cognitive processing speed in caregivers." *Gerontologist* 49 (2009): 12–22.

*Dr. Robert Sapolsky of Stanford University has shown that chronic stress:* Sorrells, S. F., et al. "The stressed CNS: When glucocorticoids aggravate inflammation." *Neuron* 64 (2009): 33–39.

*Researchers at the University of Wisconsin are finding that:* Shackman, A. J., et al. "Stress potentiates early and attenuates late stages of visual processing." *J Neurosci* 31: 1156–61.

*Studies show that after several days of cortisol injections:* Newcomer, J. W., et al. "Decreased memory performance in healthy humans induced by stress-level cortisol treatment." *Arch Gen Psychiatry* 56 (1999): 527–33.

*other recent studies indicate that when we're under stress, some forms of emotional memory may actually improve:* Buchanan, T. W., and W. R. Lovallo. "Enhanced memory for emotional material following stress-level cortisol treatment in humans." *Psychoneuroendocrinology* 26 (2001): 307–17.

*When scientists measure a volunteer's blood markers of inflammation:* Simpson, N., and D. F. Dinges. "Sleep and inflammation." *Nutr Rev* 65 (2007): S244–52.

*Dr. Wendy Troxel and colleagues at the University of Pittsburgh have found that people with sleep problems:* Troxel, W. M., et al. "Sleep symptoms predict the development of the metabolic syndrome." *Sleep* 33 (2010): 1633–40.

*During sleep our brain's memory centers are busy working:* Stickgold, R. "Sleep-dependent memory consolidation." *Nature* 437 (2005): 1272–78.

*About 30 percent of people suffer from insomnia:* Morin, C. M., et al. "Epidemiology of insomnia: prevalence, self-help treatments, consultations, and determinants of help-seeking behaviors." *Sleep Med* 7 (2006): 123–30.

*Dr. David Meyer and associates at the University of Michigan:* Rubinstein, J. S., et al. "Executive control of cognitive processes in task switching." *J Exp Psychol Hum Percept Perform* 27 (2001): 763–97.

*Dr. Britta Hölzel and associates at Harvard Medical School recently put:* Hölzel, B. K., et al. "Mindfulness practice leads to increases in regional brain gray matter density." *Psychiatry Res: Neuroimaging* 191 (2011): 36–42.

*Meditation also fires up the frontal areas of the brain:* Davanger, S., et al. "Meditation-specific prefrontal cortical activation during acem meditation: an fMRI study." *Percept Mot Skills* 111 (2010): 291–306.

Newberg, A. B., et al. "Meditation effects on cognitive function and cerebral blood flow in subjects with memory loss: A preliminary study." *J Alzheim Dis* 20 (2010): 517–26.

*After just three months of meditation training, volunteers became better able to release:* Slagter, H. A., et al. "Mental training affects distribution of limited brain resources." *PLoS Biol* 5(6): e138. doi:10.1371/journal.pbio.0050138.

*A recent UCLA study found that anticipated rejection:* Slavich, G. M., et al. "Neural sensitivity to social rejection is associated with inflammatory responses to social stress." *Proc Natl Acad Sci USA* 2011. www.pnas.org/cgi/doi/10.1073/pnas.1009164107.

*Tai chi helps reduce fatigue and pain:* Wang, C., et al. "A randomized trial of tai chi for fibromyalgia." *N Engl J Med* 363 (2010): 743–54.

*Researchers at the Chinese University in Hong Kong:* Lam, L. C., et al. "Interim follow-up of a randomized controlled trial comparing Chinese style mind body (Tai Chi) and stretching exercises on cognitive function in subjects at risk of progressive cognitive decline." *Int J Geriatr Psychiatry* 26 (2011): 733–40.

*Dr. Michael Irwin and colleagues at UCLA have demonstrated that tai chi:* Irwin, M. R., et al. "Major depressive disorder and immunity to Varicella-Zoster virus in the elderly." *Brain Behav Immun* 25 (2011): 759–66.

*Nearly 10 percent of the population suffers from some form of social anxiety:* Stein, M. B., et al. "A prospective community study of adolescents and young adults." *Arch Gen Psychiatry* 58 (2001): 251–56.

Bryant, C., et al. "The prevalence of anxiety in older adults: Methodological issues and a review of the literature." *J Aff Disord* 109 (2008): 233–50.

*Functional MRI studies have shown that humor:* Goldin, P. R., et al. "The neural bases of amusement and sadness: A comparison of block contrast and subject-specific emotion intensity regression approaches." *NeuroImage* 27 (2005): 26–36.

*Despite the lingering stigma of psychotherapy and psychiatric treatment:* Leichsenring, F., and S. Rabung. "Effectiveness of long-term psychodynamic psychotherapy: A meta-analysis." *JAMA* 300 (2008): 1551–65.

## CHAPTER 8

*A recent survey from the Alzheimer's Foundation of America:* Alzheimer's Foundation of America Survey. "Americans with Memory Concerns Fall Short of Talking to Doctors." www.alzfdn.org/MediaCenter/073008.html.

*The Pew Internet & American Life Project:* Fox, S. "Online health search 2006." Pew Internet & American Life Project. October 29, 2006. www.pewinternet.org/Reports/2006/Online-Health-Search-2006.aspx.

*The goal is to partner with your doctor:* Kasper, J., et al. "Turning signals into meaning: 'Shared decision making' meets communication theory." *Health Expect* 2011. doi: 10.1111/j.1369-7625.2011.00657.x.

*When doctors proactively involve patients in clinical decisions:* Elwyn, G., et al. "Achieving involvement: Process outcomes from a cluster randomized trial of shared decision making skill development and use of risk communication aids in general practice." *Fam Pract* 21 (2004): 337–46.

*Hypertension and diabetes sometimes lead to tiny strokes:* Schwartz, E., et al. "Cardiovascular risk factors affect hippocampal microvasculature in early AD." *Transl Neurosci* 1 (2010): 292–99.

*Our UCLA research group used functional MRI scanning:* Braskie, M. N., et al. "Vascular health risks and fMRI activation during a memory task in older adults." *Neurobiol Aging* 31 (2010): 1532–42.

*A study of more than 1,300 older hypertensive volunteers:* Godin, O., et al. "Antihypertensive treatment and change in blood pressure are associated with the progression of white matter lesion volumes: The Three-City (3C)-Dijon Magnetic Resonance Imaging Study." *Circulation* 123 (2011): 266–73.

*People with mild cognitive impairment who receive treatment for diabetes, high blood pressure:* Li, J., et al. "Vascular risk factors promote conversion from mild cognitive impairment to Alzheimer disease." *Neurology* 76 (2011): 1485–91.

*Researchers at Johns Hopkins in Baltimore found that for people age 60:* Lin, F. R., et al. "Hearing loss and incident dementia." *Arch Neurol* 68 (2011): 214–20.

*Dr. Christine Reitz and coworkers at Columbia:* Reitz, C., et al. "Association of higher levels of high-density lipoprotein cholesterol in elderly individuals and lower risk of late-onset Alzheimer disease." *Arch Neurol* 67 (2010): 1491–97.

*A wide range of physical conditions also can contribute to memory loss:* Small, G. W., and L. F. Jarvik. "The dementia syndrome." *Lancet* 2 (1982): 1443–46.

*Although the use of statin drugs in people with high cholesterol levels:* Bettermann, K., et al. "Statins, risk of dementia, and cognitive function: Secondary analysis of the Ginkgo Evaluation of Memory Study." *J Stroke Cerebrovasc Dis* 12 Jan 2011.

*New research has found that the insulin used to treat diabetes:* De Felice, F. G., et al. "Protection of synapses against Alzheimer's-linked toxins: Insulin signaling prevents the pathogenic binding of Aβ oligomers." *Proc Natl Acad Sci USA* 106 (2009): 1971–76.

*A recent study that included more than 13,000 volunteers:* Szekely, C. A., et al. "No Advantage of Aβ42-lowering NSAIDs for prevention of Alzheimer dementia in six pooled cohort studies." *Neurology* 70 (2008): 2291–98.

*An estimated 50 percent or more of adults take vitamins:* Radimer, K., et al. "Dietary supplement use by US adults: data from the National Health and Nutrition Examination Survey, 1999–2000." *Am J Epidemiol* 160 (2004): 339–49.

Small, G. W. "Beyond standard anti-dementia therapies: Diet, exercise, socialization, and supplements." *CNS Spectrums* 13 (Suppl 16) (2008): 31–33.

*Research from Nizam's Institute of Medical Sciences:* Usharani, P., et al. "Effect of NCB-02, atorvastatin and placebo on endothelial function, oxidative stress and inflammatory markers in patients with type 2 diabetes mellitus: A randomized, parallel-group, placebo-controlled, 8-week study." *Drugs R D* 9 (2008): 243–50.

*Controlled studies using phosphatidylserine supplements have demonstrated:* Hubbard, W. K. "Letter updating the phosphatidylserine and cognitive function and dementia qualified health claim." FDA, U.S. Department of Health and Human Services. November 24, 2004. www.fda.gov/Food/LabelingNutrition/LabelClaims/Qualified HealthClaims/ucm072993.htm.

*A recent double-blind study from Sourasky Medical Center:* Vakhapova, V., et al. "Phosphatidylserine containing omega-3 fatty acids may improve memory abilities in non-demented elderly with memory complaints: A double-blind placebo-controlled trial." *Dement Geriatr Cogn Disord* 29 (2010): 467–74.

*Japanese investigators used soybean-derived:* Kato-Kataoka, A., et al. "Soybean-derived phosphatidylserine improves memory function of the elderly Japanese subjects with memory complaints." *J Clin Biochem Nutr* 47 (2010): 246–55.

*Folate, or folic acid (an antioxidant B vitamin), is recommended during pregnancy:* Honein, M. A., et al. "Impact of folic acid fortification of the US food supply on the occurrence of neural tube defects." *JAMA* 285 (2001): 2981–86.

*These two B vitamins as well as vitamin $B_6$ are involved in the breakdown of homocysteine:* Hooshmand. B., et al. "Homocysteine and holotranscobalamin and the risk of Alzheimer disease: A longitudinal study." *Neurology* 75 (2010): 1408–14.

Riggs, K. M., et al. "Relations of vitamin B-12, vitamin B-6, folate, and homocysteine to cognitive performance in the Normative Aging Study." *Am J Clin Nutr* 63 (1996): 306–14.

*Oxford University investigators:* Smith, A. D., et al. "Homocysteine-lowering by B vitamins slows the rate of accelerated brain atrophy in mild cognitive impairment: A randomized controlled trial." *PLoS One* 5 (2010): e12244.

*vitamin $B_{12}$ may help the body control inflammation:* Politis, A., et al. "Vitamin B12 levels in Alzheimer's disease: association with clinical features and cytokine production." *J Alzheim Dis* 19 (2010): 481–88.

*Vitamin D not only keeps our bones strong:* Iwamoto, J., et al. "Prevention of hip fractures by exposure to sunlight and pharmacotherapy in patients with Alzheimer's disease." *Aging Clin Exp Res* 21 (2009): 277–81.

Annweiler, C., et al. "Vitamin D and ageing: Neurological issues." *Neuropsychobiology* 62 (2010): 139–50.

*Low levels of vitamin D are associated:* Llewellyn, D. J., et al. "Vitamin D and risk of cognitive decline in elderly persons." *Arch Intern Med* 170 (2010): 1135–41.

*In a study of more than 5,000 older women:* Annweiler, C., et al. "Dietary intake of vitamin D and cognition in older women: a large population-based study." *Neurology* 75 (2010): 1810–16.

*In the late 1990s Dr. Mary Sano:* Sano, M., et al. "A controlled trial of selegiline, alpha-tocopherol, or both as treatment for Alzheimer's disease." *N Engl J Med* 336 (1997): 1216–22.

*Dr. Edgar Miller and colleagues:* Miller, E. R., et al. "Meta-analysis: High-dosage vitamin E supplementation may increase all-cause mortality." *Ann Int Med* 142 (2005): 37–46.

*Studies of antioxidant supplements:* Devore, E. E., et al. "Dietary antioxidants and long-term risk of dementia." *Arch Neurol* 67 (2010): 819–25.

Gray, S. L., et al. "Antioxidant vitamin supplement use and risk of dementia or Alzheimer's disease in older adults." *J Am Geriatr Soc* 56 (2008): 291–95.

*Ginkgo biloba's antioxidant and brain circulation properties:* DeKosky, S. T., et al. "Ginkgo biloba for prevention of dementia: A randomized controlled trial." *JAMA* 300 (2008): 2253–62.

*Docosahexaenoic acid (DHA):* Lopez, L. B., et al. "High dietary and plasma levels of the omega-3 fatty acid docosahexaenoic acid are associated with decreased dementia risk: the Rancho Bernardo study." *J Nutr Health Aging* 15 (2011): 25–31.

Quinn, J. F., et al. "Docosahexaenoic acid supplementation and cognitive decline in Alzheimer disease: A randomized trial." *JAMA* 304 (2010): 1903–11.

*using a form of American ginseng:* Scholey, A., et al. "Effects of American ginseng (Panax quinquefolius) on neurocognitive function: An acute, randomised, double-blind, placebo-controlled, crossover study." *Psychopharmacology* 212 (2010): 345–56.

Geng, J., et al. "Ginseng for cognition." *Cochrane Database Syst Rev* 8 Dec 2010. 12:CD007769.

*Because an Alzheimer's brain is deficient in acetylcholine:* Small, G. W. "Alzheimer's disease and other dementing disorders," in *Comprehensive Textbook of Psychiatry*, 9th ed., B. J. and V. A. Sadock, eds. Williams & Wilkins: Baltimore, 2009, pp. 4058–65.

*One study of mild cognitive impairment found that patients taking donepezil:* Petersen, R. C., et al. "Vitamin E and donepezil for the treatment of mild cognitive impairment." *N Engl J Med* 352 (2005): 2379–88.

*Despite such mixed results from controlled clinical trials:* Schneider, L. S., et al. "Treatment with cholinesterase inhibitors and memantine of patients in the Alzheimer's Disease Neuroimaging Initiative." *Arch Neurol* 68 (2011): 58–66.

*adults with only mild memory complaints who took donepezil for 18 months:* Silverman, D.H.S., et al. "Long-term effects of donepezil versus placebo on regional brain metabolism in minimally impaired subjects." Alzheimer's Association International Conference on Alzheimer's Disease (ICAD), 2008.

*Dr. Steven Ferris and colleagues at New York University:* Ferris, S., et al. "A double-blind, placebo-controlled trial of memantine in age-associated memory impairment (memantine in AAMI)." *Int J Geriatr Psychiatry* 22 (2007): 448–55.

*Dr. Ralph Nixon and colleagues at the Nathan Kline Institute:* Nixon, R. A., and D. S. Yang. "Autophagy failure in Alzheimer's disease: locating the primary defect." *Neurobiol Dis* 3 Feb 2011.

*correlation between the age of Down syndrome:* Nelson, L. D., et al. "PET of brain amyloid and tau in adults with Down syndrome." *Arch Neurol* 68 (2001): 768–74.

*Investigators from UCLA's Alzheimer's Disease Research Center recently found that depression:* Lu, P. H., et al. "Donepezil delays progression to AD in MCI subjects with depressive symptoms." *Neurology* 72 (2009): 2115–21.

*Investigators at the Rotman Research Institute:* Mayberg, H. S. "Modulating dysfunctional limbic-cortical circuits in depression: Towards development of brain-based algorithms for diagnosis and optimised treatment." *Br Med Bull* 65 (2003): 193–207.

## CHAPTER 9

*According to a recent study published in the* European Journal of Social Psychology: Lally, P., et al. "How are habits formed: Modelling habit formation in the real world." *Eur J Soc Psychol* 40 (2010): 998–1009.

*When people grasp the connection between how their lifestyle:* Sarkisian, C. A., et al. "Pilot test of an attribution retraining intervention to raise walking levels in sedentary older adults." *J Am Geriatr Soc* 55 (2007): 1842–46.

*Neuroscientists have been able to pinpoint brain regions:* Lang, P. J., et al. "Emotion, motivation, and anxiety: Brain mechanisms and psychophysiology." *Biol Psychiatry* 44 (1998): 1248–63.

Savine, A. C., and T. S. Braver. "Motivated cognitive control: Reward incentives modulate preparatory neural activity during task-switching." *J Neurosci* 30 (2010): 10, 294–305.
*Your posture affects both your physical and mental state:* Dijkstra, K., et al. "Body posture facilitates retrieval of autobiographical memories." *Cognition* 102 (2007): 139–49.
*Remember, a ten-minute conversation is a better brain booster than watching:* Ybarra, O., et al. "Mental exercising through simple socializing: Social interaction promotes general cognitive functioning." *Pers Soc Psychol Bull* 34 (2008): 248–59.

## CHAPTER 10

*Dr. Catherine Sarkisian:* Sarkisian, C. A., et al. "Pilot test of an attribution retraining intervention to raise walking levels in sedentary older adults." *J Am Geriatr Soc* 55 (2007): 1842–46.
*why the Alzheimer's prevention program appears to be so effective:* Pope, S. K., et al. "Will a healthy lifestyle help prevent Alzheimer's disease?" *Ann Rev Public Health* 42 (2003): 111–32.
*Investigators at the University of Pittsburgh found:* Yang, K., et al. "Outcomes of health care providers' recommendations for healthy lifestyle among U.S. adults with prediabetes." *Metab Syndr Relat Disord* 9 (2011): 231–37.
*Claire Adams of Louisiana State University:* Adams, C. E., and M. R. Leary. "Promoting self-compassionate attitudes toward eating among restrictive and guilty eaters." *J Soc Clin Psych* 26 (2007): 1120–44.
*Systematic research has found that when people gain confidence:* Sol, B. G., et al. "The effect of self-efficacy on cardiovascular lifestyle." *Eur J Cardiovasc Nurs* 29 Jul 2010. www.sciencedirect.com/science/article/pii/S1474515110000812.
*Research on self-monitoring shows that:* Yon, B. A., et al. "Personal digital assistants are comparable to traditional diaries for dietary self-monitoring during a weight loss program." *J Behav Med* 30 (2007): 165–75.
Burke, L. E., et al. "Self-monitoring in weight loss: A systematic review of the literature." *J Am Diet Assoc* 111 (2011): 92–102.

## Q&A

*Is it true that people whose mothers:* Honea, R. A., et al. "Reduced gray matter volume in normal adults with a maternal family history of Alzheimer disease." *Neurology* 74 (2010): 113–20.
Mosconi, L., et al. "Declining brain glucose metabolism in normal individuals with a maternal history of Alzheimer disease." *Neurology* 72 (2009): 513–20.
*I have heard that some people have their dental fillings replaced or removed:* Kamer, A. R., et al. "Inflammation and Alzheimer's disease: Possible role of periodontal diseases." *Alzheim Dement* 4 (2008): 242–50.
Bates, M. N. "Mercury amalgam dental fillings: An epidemiologic assessment." *Int J Hyg Environ Health* 209 (2006): 309–16.
*Do women have a greater risk for dementia:* Ruitenberg, A., et al. "Incidence of dementia: Does gender make a difference?" *Neurobiol Aging* 22 (2001): 575–80.
*I know that severe head trauma can cause brain injury, but how bad does it have to be to increase your risk for Alzheimer's?:* Kumar, V., and L. J. Kinsella. "Healthy brain aging:

Effect of head injury, alcohol and environmental toxins." *Clin Geriatr Med* 26 (2010): 29–44.

Matser, E .J., et al. "Neuropsychological impairment in amateur soccer players." *JAMA* 282 (1999): 9071–73.

***Does any kind of exercise help keep your brain healthy or do I have to do power walks:*** Voss, M. W., et al. "Plasticity of brain networks in a randomized intervention trial of exercise training in older adults." *Front Aging Neurosci* 2 (2010): 1–17.

***I heard that cooking with aluminum pots:*** Frisardi, V., et al. "Aluminum in the diet and Alzheimer's disease: From current epidemiology to possible disease-modifying treatment." *J Alzheim Dis* 20 (2010): 17–30.

Rondeau, V., et al. "Aluminum and silica in drinking water and the risk of Alzheimer's disease or cognitive decline: Findings from 15-year follow-up of the PAQUID cohort." *Am J Epidemiol* 169 (2009): 489–96.

***I've been overweight most of my life and finally saw a nutritionist who helped me lose 30 pounds:*** Gunsted, J., et al. "Improved memory function 12 weeks after bariatric surgery." *Surg Obes Rel Dis* 30 Oct 2010.

Brinkworth, G. D., et al. "Long-term effects of a very low-carbohydrate diet and a low-fat diet on mood and cognitive function." *Arch Intern Med* 169 (2009): 1873–80.

***If I train my memory, will I become more intelligent?:*** Jaeggi, S. M., et al. "Short- and long-term benefits of cognitive training." *Proc Natl Acad Sci U S A* 108 (2011):10,081–86.

***People are always talking about cell phones causing brain tumors:*** Volkow, N. D., et al. "Effects of cell phone radiofrequency signal exposure on brain glucose metabolism." *JAMA* 305 (2011): 808–13.

***I've heard that cellphones may protect my brain:*** Arendash, G. W., T. Mori, et al. "Electromagnetic field treatment protects against and reverses cognitive impairment in Alzheimer's disease mice." *J Alzheim Dis* 19 (2010): 191–210.

***I'm confused by what I've heard in the news about estrogen replacement therapy:*** Whitmer, R. A., et al. "Timing of hormone therapy and dementia: The critical window theory revisited." *Ann Neurol* 69 (2011): 163–69.

***My doctor says I don't have Alzheimer's, but I wonder if I should start taking an anti-Alzheimer's drug:*** Petersen, R. C., et al. "Vitamin E and donepezil for the treatment of mild cognitive impairment." *N Engl J Med* 352 (2005): 2379–88.

Silverman, D.H.S., et al. "Long-term effects of donepezil versus placebo on regional brain metabolism in minimally impaired subjects." Alzheimer's Association International Conference on Alzheimer's Disease, 2008.

***I know smoking can give a person lung cancer:*** Cataldo, J. K., et al. "Cigarette smoking is a risk factor for Alzheimer's Disease: an analysis controlling for tobacco industry affiliation." *J Alzheim Dis* 19 (2010): 465–80.

***I know someone who smoked a lot of marijuana:*** Yücel, M., et al. "Regional brain abnormalities associated with long-term heavy cannabis use." *Arch Gen Psychiatry* 65 (2008): 694–701.

Scholes, K. E., and M. T. Martin-Iverson. "Cannabis use and neuropsychological performance in healthy individuals and patients with schizophrenia." *Psychol Med* 40 (2010): 1635–46.

Morgan, C. J., et al. "Impact of cannabidiol on the acute memory and psychotomimetic effects of smoked cannabis: Naturalistic study." *Br J Psychiatry* 197 (2010): 285–90.

*I have been taking a statin drug to lower my cholesterol:* Bettermann, K., et al. "Statins, risk of dementia, and cognitive function: Secondary analysis of the Ginkgo Evaluation of Memory Study." *J Stroke Cerebrovasc Dis* 12 Jan 2011. www.sciencedirect.com/science/article/pii/S1052305710002533.

McGuinness, B., et al. "Statins for the treatment of dementia." *Cochrane Database Syst Rev* 14 Aug 2010 (8): CD007514.

Evans, M. A., and B. A. Golomb. "Statin-associated adverse cognitive effects: Survey results from 171 patients." *Pharmacotherapy* 29 (2009): 800–11.

*I just read about some kind of new nasal spray that's supposed to protect you from getting Alzheimer's disease:* Lifshitz, V., et al. "Immunotherapy of cerebrovascular amyloidosis in a transgenic mouse model." *Neurobiol Aging* 1 Mar 2011. www.sciencedirect.com/science/article/pii/S019745801100008X.

*I recently read that a medicine used to prevent kidney transplant rejection has been shown to stop Alzheimer's disease:* Caccamo, A., et al. "Molecular interplay between mammalian target of rapamycin (mTOR), amyloid-beta, and Tau: Effects on cognitive impairments." *J Biol Chem* 185 (2010): 13,107–120.

## BONUS CHAPTER

*Is it true that a new cancer drug is being tested:* Zhang, B., et al. "The microtubule-stabilizing agent, epothilone D, reduces axonal dysfunction, neurotoxicity, cognitive deficits, and Alzheimer-like pathology in an interventional study with aged tau transgenic mice." *J Neurosci* 32 (2012): 3601–11.

*I heard that some scientists discovered that Alzheimer's spreads:* Nath, S., et al: "Spreading of neurodegenerative pathology via neuron-to-neuron transmission of β-amyloid." *J Neurosci* 32 (2012): 8767–77.

*A coworker told me that diabetes doubles the risk for getting Alzheimer's disease:* Ohara, T., et al. "Glucose tolerance status and risk of dementia in the community: The Hisayama Study." *Neurology* 77 (2011): 1126–34.

*Is it true that air pollution can speed up mental decline:* Wellenius, G. A., et al. "Ambient air pollution and the risk of acute ischemic stroke." *Arch Intern Med* 172 (2012): 229–34.

*I read somewhere that eating fish can make your brain larger:* RSNA Press Release, Nov. 30, 2011, www2.rsna.org/timssnet/media/pressreleases/pr_target.cfm?id=571.

Tan, Z. S., et al. "Red blood cell ω-3 fatty acid levels and markers of accelerated brain aging." *Neurology* 78 (2012): 658–64.

*I saw on TV that doctors had used electric probes:* Smith, G. S., et al. "Increased cerebral metabolism after 1 year of deep brain stimulation in Alzheimer's disease." *Arch Neurol* 2012, May 7. [Epub ahead of print].

*Everyone is talking about an impending Alzheimer's epidemic:* Alzheimer's Association. *2012 Alzheimer's Disease Facts and Figures.* Available online: www.alz.org/downloads/facts_figures_2012.pdf.

Barnes, D. E., and K. Yaffe. "The projected effect of risk factor reduction on Alzheimer's disease prevalence." *Lancet Neurol* 10 (2011): 819–28.

*I have been tested and found out I have a genetic risk:* Head, D., et al. "Exercise engagement as a moderator of the effects of APOE genotype on amyloid deposition." *Arch Neurol* 69 (2012): 636–43.

*I read that scientists have discovered special immune proteins:* Ostrowitzki, S., et al. "Mechanism of amyloid removal in patients with Alzheimer disease treated with gantenerumab." *Arch Neurol* 69 (2012): 198–207.

*Lots of people I know have started drinking coconut oil:* Newport, M. T., and C. Hirsch. *Alzheimer's Disease: What If There Was a Cure?* Laguna Beach, CA: Basic Health, 2011.

Granholm, A. C., et al. "Effects of a saturated fat and high cholesterol diet on memory and hippocampal morphology in the middle-aged rat." *J Alzheimers Dis* 14 (2008): 133–45.

*I'm becoming addicted to playing* **Angry Birds**: Boot, W. R., et al. "The effects of video game playing on attention, memory, and executive control." *Acta Psychol* 129 (2008): 387–98.

*I was taking a lot of over-the-counter herbs:* Cupp, M. J. "Herbal remedies: Adverse effects and drug interactions." *Am Fam Physician* 59 (1999): 1239–44.

Grossberg, G. T., and B. Fox. *The Essential Herb-Drug-Vitamin Interaction Guide: The Safe Way to Use Medications and Supplements Together.* New York: Broadway Books, 2007.

*I know that a good night's sleep improves my mental focus:* Huang, Y., et al. "Effects of age and amyloid deposition on Aβ dynamics in the human central nervous system." *Arch Neurol* 69 (2012): 51–8.

# List of Abbreviations

*Acta Neuropathol* — *Acta Neuropathologica*

*Adv Exp Med Biol* — *Advances in Experimental Medicine and Biology*

*Aging Clin Exp Res* — *Aging Clinical and Experimental Research*

*Alzheim Dement* — *Alzheimer's & Dementia*

*Am Diet Assoc* — *American Dietetic Association*

*Am J Cardio* — *The American Journal of Cardiology*

*Am J Clin Nutr* — *The American Journal of Clinical Nutrition*

*Am J Epidemiol* — *American Journal of Epidemiology*

*Am J Geriatr Psychiatry* — *American Journal of Geriatric Psychiatry*

*Am J Med* — *The American Journal of Medicine*

*Ann Int Med* — *Annals of Internal Medicine*

*Ann Neurol* — *Annals of Neurology*

*Annu Rev Public Health* — *Annual Review of Public Health*

*Arch Gen Psychiatry* — *Archives of General Psychiatry*

*Arch Intern Med* — *Archives of Internal Medicine*

*Arch Neurol* — *Archives of Neurology*

*Behav Med* — *Behavioral Medicine*

*Biol Psychiatry* — *Biological Psychiatry*

*BMC Neurosci* — *BioMed Central Neuroscience*

*Br J Clin Pharmacol* – *British Journal of Clinical Pharmacology*

*Br J Psychiatry* — *British Journal of Psychiatry*

*Br Med Bull* — *British Medical Bulletin*

*Brain* — *Brain: A Journal of Neurology*

*Brain Behav Immun* — *Brain, Behavior, and Immunity*

*Brain Res* — *Brain Research*

*Clin Geriatr Med* — *Clinics in Geriatric Medicine*

*Clin Nurs Res* — *Clinical Nursing Research*

*Cochrane Database Syst Rev* — *Cochrane Database Systematic Reviews*

*Contemp Longterm Care* — *Contemporary Long Term Care*

*Crit Rev Food Sci Nutr* — *Critical Reviews in Food Science and Nutrition*

*Dement Geriatr Cogn Disord* — *Dementia and Geriatric Cognitive Disorders*

*Drugs R D* — *Drugs in R&D*

*Eur J Cardiovasc Nurs* — *European Journal of Cardiovascular Nursing*

*Eur J Hum Genet* — *European Journal of Human Genetics*

*Eur J Neurol* — *European Journal of Neurology*

*Eur J Soc Psychol* — *European Journal of Social Psychology*

*Expert Rev Neurother* — *Expert Reviews of Neurotherapeutics*

*Fam Pract* — *Family Practice*

*FASEB J* — *The Journal of the Federation of American Societies for Experimental Biology*

*Food Chem Toxicol* — *Food and Chemical Toxicology*

*Front Aging Neurosci* — *Frontiers in Aging Neuroscience*

*Health Expect* — *Health Expectations*

*Int J Hyg Environ Health* — *International Journal of Hygiene and Environmental Health*

*Int J Geriatr Psychiatry* — *International Journal of Geriatric Psychiatry*

*Int J Obes — International Journal of Obesity (London)*
*Int J Obesity Relat Metab Disord — International Journal of Obesity and Related Metabolic Disorders*
*Int Psychogeriatr — International Psychogeriatrics*
*Int J Women Health — International Journal of Women's Health*
*J Aff Disord — Journal of Affective Disorders*
*J Aging Phys Act — Journal of Aging and Physical Activity*
*J Alzheim Dis — Journal of Alzheimer's Disease*
*J Am Coll Nutrition — Journal of the American College of Nutrition*
*J Am Diet Assoc — Journal of the American Dietetic Association*
*J Am Geriatr Soc — Journal of the American Geriatrics Society*
*JAMA — Journal of the American Medical Association*
*J Biol Chem — Journal of Biological Chemistry*
*J Clin Biochem Nutr — Journal of Clinical Biochemistry and Nutrition*
*J Clin Endocrinol Metab — Journal of Clinical Endocrinology & Metabolism*
*J Consumer Res — Journal of Consumer Research*
*J Epidemiol Community Health — Journal of Epidemiology and Community Health*
*J Exp Psychol Hum Percept Perform — Journal of Experimental Psychology: Human Perception and Performance*
*J Gerontol A Biol Sci Med Sci — Journal of Gerontology Series A: Biological Sciences Medical Science*
*J Int Med — Journal of Internal Medicine*
*J Neurochem — Journal of Neurochemistry*
*J Neurosci — Journal of Neuroscience*
*J Strength Cond Res — Journal of Strength and Conditioning Research*
*J Neurobiol — Journal of Neurobiology*
*J Nutr Health Aging — Journal of Nutritional Health and Aging*
*J Stroke Cerebrovasc Dis — Journal of Stroke and Cerebrovascular Diseases*
*Lancet Neurol — The Lancet: Neurology*
*Med J Aust — The Medical Journal of Australia*
*Metab Syndr Relat Disord — Metabolic Syndrome and Related Disorders*
*Mini Rev Med Chem — Mini-Reviews in Medicinal Chemistry*
*N Engl J Med — New England Journal of Medicine*
*Nat Med —Nature Medicine*
*Nat Rev Drug Discov — Nature Reviews Drug Discovery*
*Neurobiol Aging — Neurobiology of Aging*
*Neurobiol Dis — Neurobiology of Disease*
*Neuroepidemiol — Neuroepidemiology*
*Neurosci Res Program Bull — Neurosciences Research Program Bulletin*
*NIH Consens State Sci Statements — National Institutes of Health Consensus on State-of-the-Science Statements*
*Nutr Neurosci — Nutritional Neuroscience*
*Nutr Rev — Nutrition Reviews*
*Percept Mot Skills — Perceptual and Motor Skills*

*PLoS Biol — Public Library of Science: Biology*
*Pers Soc Psychol Bull — Personality and Social Psychology Bulletin*
*Proc Natl Acad Sci USA — Procedures of the National Academy of Sciences of the United States of America*
*Prostaglandins Leukot Essent Fatty Acids — Prostaglandins, Leukotrienes & Essential Fatty Acids*
*Psychiatry Res: Neuroimaging — Psychiatry Research: Neuroimaging*
*Psychol Med — Psychological Medicine*
*Psychosom Med — Psychosomatic Medicine*
*Sleep Med — Sleep Medicine*
*Surg Obes Rel Dis — Surgery for Obesity and Related Diseases*
*Transl Neurosci — Translational Neuroscience*

# Index

inflammation, 16, 17, 94, 227
  anti-inflammatory drugs, 17–19, 162
  curry, anti-inflammatory benefits,
    106–107, 165–166
  hormones damaging to brain
    by aggravating chronic
    inflammatory response, 140–141
  sleep, anti-inflammatory effect of, 143
  and vitamin B, 166–167
information overload, 141
insomnia. *See* sleep and insomnia
insula, area of brain, 92
insulin, 90, 162
  *See also* diabetes
Internet. *See* online information
irritation
  and coffee consumption, 104
  symptom of stress, 139
isometric exercises, 80–81

## J, K

Johns Hopkins, 161
Kansas State University, 93
kidney transplant rejection, medicine
  used to prevent, 175
kitchen, stocking, 180–182
knee joints, strengthening, 76

## L

language
  foreign-language speakers, avoidance
    of Alzheimer's disease, 116
  tip-of-the-tongue phenomenon, 2,
    54, 62–63, 228
  vocabulary improvements during
    middle age, 51

laughter and humor, correlation with
  degree of brain activity, 152
lawn mowing, 77
learning, within memory, 47, 163
  brain recruits neighboring circuits to
    solve tasks, 53
left brain *vs.* right brain function, 35,
    52, 114–117
Lewy body dementia, 170
lifestyle changes. *See* habits and habit-
  forming behavior
listening, skills enhancement, 200
lobster, 101
loneliness/dementia connection, 115
long-term memory, 6, 48, 50, 51
*LOOK, SNAP, CONNECT* strategy,
    54–65, 227, 228
  in daily routine, 245, 246
  and the story method, 52
  training for first seven days, 184–220
lost items. *See* misplaced items
Louisiana State University, 231
lunches, first seven days, 183–220
lycopene, 98
lysosomes to degrade and process
  waste proteins, 173

## M

MacArthur Study of Successful Aging,
    14
mackerel, 169
maintaining healthy lifestyle changes,
    223–235
malleability of brain, 52, 111
Mantle, Mickey, quotation by, 154
marijuana use, effect of, 168
Mayo Clinic, 10

puzzles and mental games to improve
brain health, 111–113, 117–119
*See also* mental workouts

## Q

quad stretch, 85
questions and answers, 238–244,
271–274
quick positive results, 24
quinoa, 180

## R

racquet sports, 77
raking leaves, 77
RAND Corporation, 21
Rapamune (rapamycin), 175
Razadyne (galantamine), 170
reading
as brain exercise, 112–113, 163
causing insomnia, 144
recall, within memory, 47
brain recruiting neighboring circuits
for, 53
cholinergic neurotransmitters, 163
recalling names, 46
recent research and studies regarding
Alzheimer's disease treatment,
238–244
red meat, 89
references, 256–274
relaxation strategies, 149
*See also* stress management
repair of damaged cells *vs.* protection
of healthy brain ones, 231
research study participation.
*See* clinical trials

resistance training, 71
resveratrol, 103–104
right brain *vs.* left brain function, 35,
52, 114–117
rivastigmine (Exelon), 170
Roman Room Method, 64–65
Rotman Research Institute, 174
Rotterdam Study, 96
Rush University Medical Center, 139

## S

Salk Institute for Biological Studies, 110
salmon, 96, 101, 169
satiation, 92
scaling hills, 76
scallops, 101
*Science* magazine, 91
scientific references, 256–274
sedentary people
starting fitness programs, effect on
brains, 70
*See also* physical fitness
self-esteem, 88
self-forgiveness, 231–232
self-indulgence, 231–232
self-inflicted stress, 151
*See also* stress management
self-monitoring, 232–235
progress charts, 250–251
SeniorNet, 254
sensory memory, 47, 48
new information, older brain's
processing of, 51
short-term memory, 6, 47, 48
new information, older brain's
processing of, 51
shrimp, 101

urinary tract infection contributing
to memory loss and mental
symptoms, 161
U.S. Department of Veterans Affairs,
254

**V**

Vanderbilt School of Medicine, 97
vascular dementia, 170
vegetables, 89, 101–102
vegetarians, pantry items, 180
visual images to recall names, 59
visualization to control cravings,
91–92
vitamins and supplements, 164–165,
231, 243, 244
herbal treatments for Alzheimer's
prevention is still limited, 169
to lower risk for Alzheimer's disease,
157, 243
multivitamin supplements, 164,
166–167
side effects, 244
vitamin B, 166–167
vitamin C, 168
vitamin D, 167, 243
vitamin E, 96, 168
vocabulary improvements during
middle age, 51

**W**

Wagner, Jane, quotation by, 136
walking, 69, 75, 76, 226
to delay onset of symptoms, 22, 23
stress management, 150
warm-ups for exercise, 75

waste material from cells, removal, 16,
143, 173
water consumption, 194
water-soluble *vs.* fat-soluble vitamins,
164
waxy plaques. *See* amyloid plaques and
tau tangles
weekly chart for tracking exercise, 250
weight control, 41, 87–88
ideal body weights, 41, 89–90
*See also* nutrition and dietary habits
weight-lifting equipment, 79
weight-loss surgery, and improved
memory, concentration, and
problem-solving abilities, 105
white matter in brain, 52, 114
wild fish *vs.* farmed fish, 101
wine, 102–104
women, increased risk in, 20
Women's Health Initiative, 162
word-finding delays, 2, 54, 62–63, 228
word pairs and word pair exercises,
55, 58
working memory, 47
worry
making memory performance
worse, 37
"the worried well," 8
*See also* stress management

**Y, Z**

Yale University, 49
yard work, 77
yoga for stress management, 150, 151
yogurt, 101–102
young brain *vs.* old brain, photo, 16
Zoloft, 72, 73